ISBN 9781092732512

Note: The no-cooking portions of this book rely, to a large extent, on off-the-shelf foods. At publication, these foods were widely available in most super-markets. But food products come and go. So if there is a frozen entrée or soup selection that is out of stock, or that's been discontinued, or perhaps you don't like, or that you forgot to pick up while shopping, please substitute another food that has **approximately** the same caloric value and nutritional content. In this regard, many dieters have found the foods listed in the Appendices at the end of this book to be helpful.

90-DAY
PERFECT DIET
1200-CALORIE

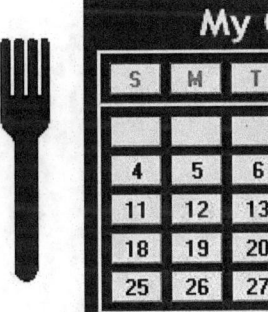

Gail Johnson, M.S.
Elena Novak

NoPaperPress™

CONTENTS

What's In This Book

Most of us are busy – extremely busy under pressure to balance career, family, finances, a social life, friends, learning, and the list goes on and on. You know you should lose weight, but your life is just too hectic to plan and prepare low-calorie meals. The *90-Day Perfect Diet* can help. For those days when you don't have the time or energy to cook, choose from **50 daily no-cooking menus**. On the weekend, or whenever you have the time to cook, select from **50 daily cooking menus** complete with delicious easy to prepare recipes. In summary then, the *90-Day Perfect Diet* features:
- **- 50 Daily No-Cooking Menus**
- **- 50 Daily Cooking Menus**
- **- 53 Recipes**

And every day on the *90-Day Perfect Diet* you get to decide to cook or not to cook and then you pick an appropriate daily menu from the large selection. But know that whether or not you cook you will be eating 1200 Calories and will lose the same amount of weight.

Why You Lose Weight

Most weight loss experts agree that when the energy value of the food you eat minus waste, equals the sum of your basal metabolic energy plus the energy you expend during physical activity, you will neither gain nor lose weight. They also agree that when you have an energy imbalance, you will either gain or lose weight. In general then:

- **Weight Maintenance** occurs when your food energy intake equals the total energy you expend in daily living. In this case your weight remains stable, i.e., you neither gain nor lose weight.

- **Weight Gain** occurs when your food energy intake is greater than the total energy you expend in daily living. In this case your body stores the extra energy as fat.

- **Weight Loss** occurs when your food energy intake is less than the total energy you expend in daily living. In this case your body converts stored fat (and in some cases muscle) into energy.

The measure of energy, whether in the form of food, physical activity, or heat, is the kilocalorie (hereafter simply called the Calorie). As mentioned previously, weight loss occurs when you eat fewer calories than the calories you use in your day-to-day living. This difference in calories is referred to as your calorie deficit. How much weight you lose depends on the magnitude of your calorie deficit. (In technical terms, **the calorie deficit, or calorie difference, is the driving force for weight change**.)

Most people on a weight-loss diet want to know how much weight they will lose – and how fast. Simple metabolic calculations make a rough estimate possible. Physiologists have long known that to lose one pound requires a deficit of approximately 3500 Calories. Therefore, if a person's total calorie deficit over time is known, their weight loss over time can be calculated. (See "**Expected Weight Loss** for Men/Women" later on this page.) **In summary, if you eat and exercise such that you have a calorie deficit you will lose weight!**

The Best Weight Loss Diets

According to the late Dr. Jean Mayer of Harvard and Tufts University's Department of Nutrition, a really good weight-loss diet must have the following three characteristics:

1) The diet must provide you with an understanding of weight control as well as the knowledge you need to reduce your weight to the desired level.

2) The diet must help you remain healthy while you are losing weight.

3) The diet must lead you to a healthier way of eating and exercising that will, in the long term, help you keep off the weight you have lost.

Why the 90-Day Perfect Diet?

Experts agree that a diet that promotes weight loss over a relatively longer time period is healthier and the weight loss is likely to be more permanent. These experts recommend you choose a nutritious diet that results in a weight loss of approximately 2 pounds per week – which amounts to about 26 pounds in 90 days. The *90-Day Perfect Diet* fits the bill! And because the *90-Day Perfect Diet* is not a fad and does not rely on gimmicks it will be as valid 10 or 20 years from now as it is today. The *90-Day Perfect Diet* is in fact a timeless diet!

Expected Weight Loss

Weight loss occurs when your food energy intake is less than the total energy you expend. This difference in calories is referred to as your calorie deficit. How much weight you lose depends on the magnitude of your calorie deficit. Physiologists have long known that to lose one pound requires a deficit of approximately 3,500 Calories. Therefore, if a person's total calorie deficit over time is known, their weight loss over time can be calculated.

On the *90-Day Perfect Diet – 1200 Calorie Edition*, **most women lose 23 to 33 pounds.** Smaller women, older women and less active women lose a bit less and larger women, younger women and more active women often lose much more.

On the *90-Day Perfect Diet – 1200 Calorie Edition*, **most men lose 35 to 45 pounds**. Smaller men, older men and less active men will lose a tad less and larger men, younger men and more active men frequently lose much more.

Exactly how much weight you will lose depends on how much you weigh, your age and your activity level. For the full story see *Weight Control - U.S. Edition* by Vincent W. Antonetti, Ph.D., also published by NoPaperPress.

Perfect Diet Info
The *90-Day Perfect Diet* contains meal plans, recipes and guidance for 60 fat-melting days! How long you stay on the diet, 10 days, 45 days, or all 90 days – depends on how much weight you want to lose. The *90-Day Perfect Diet* features:
- 50 Daily No-Cooking Menus starting on page 13.
- 50 Daily Cooking Menus starting on page 64.
- 53 Recipes & Diet Tips starting on page 114.

Before you begin any weight loss program you should, at the very least, **have a medical assessment, or exam.** Why? You need to make sure your health will allow you to lower your caloric intake and increase your physical activity. Depending on your age and state of health, the medical checkup may be as simple as a visit to a physician who is familiar with your medical history, or it may be a thorough physical exam. The physician conducting the medical exam should be made aware of and should approve the specific weight loss diet you're planning. Even though the *90-Day Perfect Diet* adheres to the United States Department of Agriculture balanced diet recommendations, the *90-Day Perfect Diet* may not be appropriate for everyone, such as individuals with illnesses such as heart disease, diabetes, food allergies, etc. Again, make sure you check with your physician before starting this diet, or any diet.

Using the Daily Menus
Let's look at No-Cooking **Daily Menu 1** on page 14. Most of the menu is obvious and easily understood. Find the line item **Soup** (see **Appendix B** on page 171) and note the soup calorie allowance is 110 Calories. Now go to **Appendix B** on page 171, which contains a list of 25 soup selections arranged from lowest to highest in calorie content. In Appendix B, scroll down until you find the 110 Calorie soup selections. There are two to choose from.

To find the frozen entrée for No-Cooking **Daily Menu 2** first note that the allotment for the Day 2 frozen entrée is 200 Calories. Now go to **Appendix D** on page 174, which contains a list of about 150 frozen entrées arranged from lowest to highest in calorie content. In Appendix D, scroll down until you find the 200 Calorie frozen entrées. The are four entrées to choose from. Incidentally, because the diet calls for a ham sandwich for lunch, choose something other than a meat entrée for dinner, such as a 200 Calorie chicken or pasta frozen entrée. Remember variety is the key to a nutritious diet!

Eat Perfectly

No single food can supply all the nutrients you need in the amounts you need. The most important factors in nutrition are variety, variety, variety! **Variety is the key to a nutritious diet.** As a means of setting strategies for food selection, the U.S. Department of Health and Human Services and the Department of Agriculture issue Dietary Guidelines every five years. The latest Dietary Guidelines describe a healthy diet as one that:
- Emphasizes fruits, vegetables, whole grains, and fat-free or low-fat milk.
- Includes fish, poultry, lean meats, beans and nuts.
- Is low in saturated fats, trans fats, cholesterol, salt (sodium) and added sugars.

The latest guidelines encourage adults to consume a variety of nutrient-dense foods and beverages within their caloric needs. The afore mentioned U.S. government agencies recommend how much should be eaten from each of the basic food groups (i.e., from the fruit group, vegetable group, grains group, meat and beans group, milk group, and oils group) to meet your caloric goal – whether you are trying to lose weight or maintain weight. All this information and more can be found in *Eat Smart - U.S. Edition* also published by NoPaperPress.

Even though most adults can get all the vitamins and minerals they need by merely consuming a variety of nutritious foods (from the fruit group, the vegetable group, the grains group, the meat and beans group, the milk group, and the oils group), many physicians recommend a daily multi-vitamin/mineral supplement – just in case you don't eat the way you should.

No-Cooking: Big-Bowl Salad

The **No-Cooking Daily Menus** feature frozen entrees. A problem with nearly all frozen entrees is that they don't contain enough veggies. The solution is to have a "Big-Bowl Salad" at dinnertime with your frozen entrée. A typical "Big-Bowl Salad" is shown in the photo on the next page.

To prepare a "Big-Bowl Salad" start with a relatively large soup bowl (with a volume of at least 24 ounces, or 3 cups). Add about 1½ cups of either green leaf lettuce, Romaine lettuce or a mesclun mix. Then add, as desired, veggies such as broccoli, celery, cucumber, onion, peppers, radish, spinach, tomato, or watercress, to make up the remaining 1½ cups, for a total of 3 cups.

8

This vegetable combination will, on average, total about 100 Calories. You will be eating a "Big-Bowl Salad" almost every day at dinnertime. Remember that variety is the key to a nutritious diet. So be sure to vary the ingredients of the salad.

Top your "Big-Bowl Salad" with <u>2 tablespoons</u> of any light salad dressing available at your local supermarket that contains no more than 25 Calories per tablespoon. See some of my favorite light salad dressings below. Your "Big-Bowl Salad" with salad dressing will cost you roughly 150 Calories but will be packed with lots of health-giving vitamins, minerals and fiber.

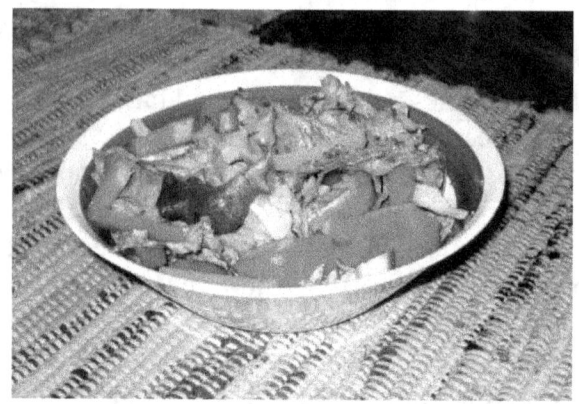

Big-Bowl Salad

Cooking: Have a Tossed Salad

One of the dinner mainstays in the **Cooking Daily Menus** is a tossed salad." To prepare your "Tossed Salad" start with a bowl that has a volume of about 16 ounces, or 2 cups. First add about 1 cup of either green leaf lettuce, Romaine lettuce or a mesclun mix. Then add at least a half cup of other veggies such as broccoli, celery, cucumber, peppers, spinach, watercress, or tomatoes. This vegetable combination will, on average, total something like 45 Calories.

You'll be eating a "Tossed Salad" just about every day at dinnertime. Once again, variety is the key to a nutritious diet. So vary the ingredients of the salad.

Top your "Tossed Salad" with <u>1½ tablespoons of any light salad dressing</u> available at your local supermarket that contains no more than 25 Calories per tablespoon.

Your "Tossed Salad" with salad dressing will cost you roughly 85 Calories but again will be packed with lots of health-giving veggies.

Our Favorite Salad Dressings

For your consideration, here are some of our favorite light salad dressings. All have a maximum of 25 Calories per tablespoon.
- **Ken's Steakhouse Fat Free Raspberry**
- **Kraft Light Done Right House Italian**
- **Wishbone Just 2 Good Honey Dijon**
- **Newman's Lighten Up Balsamic Vinaigrette**

Whole-Grain Bread

First understand that bread, more specifically whole-grain breads, are good sources of complex carbohydrates and dietary fiber, as well as several B vitamins (thiamin, riboflavin, niacin, and folate), vitamin E, and minerals (iron, magnesium and selenium). In recent years, however, sliced bread loaves have gotten larger, as have the bread slices inside these loaves. Just a few years ago the standard slice of bread contained about 65 to 70 Calories – now most are 100 plus Calories.

The *90-Day Perfect Diet* **requires whole-grain bread at 70 Calories per slice.** Quite a few bakers sell thin sliced or "light" sliced bread. The difficult part is finding a whole grain thin sliced or "light" bread (with about 70 Calories per slice). Whatever the brand, make sure the first word in the Ingredients list is "whole." "Pepperidge Farm Small Slice 100% Whole Wheat" is a good choice. It's whole grain, has 70 Calories per slice and it tastes good too.

Substituting Foods

If there is a food listed in the *90-Day Perfect Diet* that you don't like, or perhaps that you forgot to pick up while shopping, you probably can exchange or substitute another food in its place – a technique used by dieticians. For more on this go to Substituting Foods in **Appendix A** (page 167).

Important Notes

1) Coffee or tea may be caffeinated or decaf . If desired, skim milk and a sugar substitute may be added to coffee or tea. And soy or almond milk are an acceptable alternative to cow's milk.

2) Fried eggs or scrambled eggs should be cooked in a pan coated with a non-stick cooking spray. Hard-boiled eggs may be substituted for fried, scrambled or soft-boiled eggs.

3) Cereals should be whole grain and unsweetened. At the top of the list are Old-fashioned Oatmeal, Wheatena and Shredded Wheat. Among other reasonably healthy choices are Cheerios, Wheat Chex, Wheaties, some Kashi cereals and Farina. When blueberries are in season, you may **use blueberries instead of raisins** in your cereal. (Substitute ratio = 2 blueberries per raisin.)

4) Bread may be either plain or toasted whole grain, such as whole grain, whole rye or pumpernickel. Look for whole grain varieties that contain 70 Calories per slice. If desired, bread may be sprayed with a zero-calorie butter substitute. NO BUTTER!

5) When soup in a microwaveable bowl is specified, eat only one serving (8 ounces) unless otherwise noted. (Microwaveable bowls usually contain about two servings.)

6) Use freely as desired: clear unsweetened coffee, clear unsweetened tea, water, seltzer water and any diet soda, clear soups without fat, bouillon, and seasonings such as mustard, cinnamon, dill, herbs, red and black pepper, curry, vinegar, lemon juice and sections, and dill and sour pickles.

7) Use only lean cuts of meat trimmed of all visible fat. Poultry should be limited to chicken or turkey breasts (white meat only and skinless).

8) When canned tuna or salmon is specified, use only fish packed in water.

9) When the diet calls for turkey bacon, make sure the brand you buy has no more than 35 Calories per slice.

10) An unlimited amount of green salad may be eaten, but the salad dressing should be as specified.

11) If it's more convenient, any food item may be moved to any part of the day and combined with any meal or snack.

12) Although it's recommended that you follow the diet days as specified, it's fine to occasionally skip a day and/or pick and choose the days you prefer. (Nutritionally, each day stands on its own.)

13) Take a daily multi-vitamin/mineral supplement. This is important when you're on a diet – as a kind of insurance policy.

Keeping It Off

Within five years, more than 60 percent of all dieters regain every pound they have lost. Why? In most cases it's because after losing weight most people eventually revert to their pre-diet eating and exercising habits, and this inevitably leads to their regaining the weight they lost – and often more. Obviously after a diet you weigh less. The fact is the less you weigh, the less you need to eat to sustain your lower weight.

A study, published in the *Annals of Internal Medicine*, followed 4000 people for three decades suggests that in the long term, 60 percent of men and 70 percent of women will become overweight. Interestingly, half of the men and women in the study, who had made it to adulthood without a weight problem, ultimately also became overweight and a third became obese. The

point being that you can never become complacent. You must continually watch your weight because everyone is at risk of becoming overweight.

The key to long-term weight control success is knowledge and understanding, combined with desire and self-discipline. Once you reach your weight goal, we suggest you read *Weight Maintenance - U.S. Edition* by Vincent Antonetti, Ph.D. (also published by NoPaperPress) – absolutely the best weight maintenance book on the market.

NO-COOKING
Daily Meal Plans

No-Cooking Daily Menu 1

BREAKFAST	Calories	Totals
Orange juice (½ cup)	**50**	
Wheaties (¾ cup) + ½ cup skim milk + ½ banana	**190**	
Coffee (See **Notes** page 10)	**10**	**250 Cal**
SNACK		
Fresh fruit in season (apple, pear, etc)	**70**	
Coffee or tea	**10**	**80 Cal**
LUNCH		
Soup (Appendix B - page 171**)**	**110**	
Whole-grain bread (1 slice) (See page 10)	**70**	
Coffee or tea	**10**	**190 Cal**
SNACK		
Handful unsalted mixed nuts	**100**	
Coffee or tea	**10**	**110 Cal**
DINNER		
Frozen Entrée (Appendix D - page 175**)**	**290**	
"Big-Bowl Salad" (See page 8 & 10 for dressings)	**150**	
Water with lemon wedge	**15**	**465 Cal**
SNACK		
Skinny Cow Fudge Ice Cream Bar*	**110**	
Coffee or tea	**10**	**120 Cal**
* If unavailable an equivalent dessert.		**1205 Cal**

No-Cooking Daily Menu 2

BREAKFAST	Calories	Totals
Fresh or frozen strawberries (½ cup)	25	
Kashi Go Lean Waffles (2)	150	
Light Syrup (2 Tbsp)	50	
Coffee	10	235 Cal
SNACK		
Yogurt (4 oz, non-fat any flavor)	60	60 Cal
LUNCH		
Ham (2 oz) with mustard on 2 slices rye bread	300	
Fresh fruit in season (apple, peach, etc)	70	
Coffee or tea	10	380 Cal
SNACK		
Hot or ice or tea	10	10 Cal
DINNER		
Frozen Entrée (Appendix D - page 175)	200	
"Big-Bowl Salad" (See page 8)	150	
Water	0	350 Cal
SNACK		
Skinny Cow Ice Cream Sandwich*	160	
Coffee or tea	10	170 Cal
* If unavailable an equivalent dessert.		1205 Cal

No-Cooking Daily Menu 3

BREAKFAST	Calories	Totals
Grapefruit (½)	75	
Scrambled egg (Notes - page 10)	80	
Whole-grain toast (1 slice)	70	
Coffee	10	235 Cal
SNACK		
Coffee or tea	10	10 Cal
LUNCH		
Subway 6" (Turkey Breast, Cheese + veggies)*	230	
Coffee or tea	10	240 Cal
* On half of 9-grain wheat roll.		
SNACK		
Fresh fruit in season (apple, plum, etc)	70	
Coffee or tea	10	80 Cal
DINNER		
Frozen Entrée (Appendix D - page 175)	290	
"Big-Bowl Salad"	150	
Whole-grain bread (1 slice)	70	
Water with lemon wedge	15	525 Cal
SNACK		
Skinny Cow Fudge Ice Cream Bar*	110	
Coffee or tea	10	110 Cal
* If unavailable an equivalent dessert.		1200 Cal

No-Cooking Daily Menu 4

BREAKFAST	Calories	Totals
Grapefruit (½)	75	
Cheerios (1 cup) + ½ cup skim milk	160	
Coffee	10	245 Cal
SNACK		
Coffee or tea	10	10 Cal
LUNCH		
Cottage cheese (1 cup low fat)	180	
Fresh fruit in season (apple, plum, etc)	70	
Small whole-grain roll	80	
Coffee or tea	10	340 Cal
SNACK		
Coffee or tea	10	10 Cal
DINNER		
Frozen Entrée (Appendix D - page 175)	270	
"Big-Bowl Salad"	150	
Whole-grain bread (1 slice)	70	
Water	0	490 Cal
SNACK		
Handful unsalted mixed nuts	100	
Coffee or tea	10	110 Cal
		1205 Cal

No-Cooking Daily Menu 5

BREAKFAST	Calories	Totals
Cantaloupe (½ medium)	50	
Fried egg	80	
Toasted raisin bread (1 slice)	75	
Coffee	10	215 Cal
SNACK		
Yogurt (4 oz, non-fat any flavor)	60	
Coffee or tea	10	70 Cal
LUNCH		
Soup (Appendix B - page 171)*	280	
Whole-grain bread (1 slice)	70	
Hot or ice tea	0	350 Cal
* Enjoy 2 servings of a 140 Calorie soup.		
SNACK		
Banana (1 medium)	100	
Coffee or tea	10	110 Cal
DINNER		
Frozen Entrée (Appendix D - page 175)	210	
"Big-Bowl Salad"	150	
Fresh fruit in season (apple, plum, etc)	70	
Water with lemon wedge	15	445 Cal
SNACK		
Coffee or tea	10	10 Cal
		1200 Cal

No-Cooking Daily Menu 6

BREAKFAST	Calories	Totals
Tomato juice (½ cup)	20	
Shredded Wheat (1 cup) + ½ cup skim milk + ½ banana	265	
Coffee	10	295 Cal
SNACK		
Coffee or tea	10	10 Cal
LUNCH		
Chorizo, Egg & Cheese*	260	
Fresh fruit in season (peach, plum, etc)	70	
Diet soda or water	0	330 Cal
* Hot Pockets (wrap) or if unavailable an equivalent food.		
SNACK		
Coffee or tea	10	10 Cal
DINNER		
Frozen Entrée (Appendix D - page 175)	220	
"Big-Bowl Salad"	150	
Whole-grain bread (1 slice)	70	
Water	0	440 Cal
SNACK		
Popcorn Mini Bag**	110	
Coffee or tea	10	120 Cal
** Such as Orville Redenbacher's Smart Pop		1205 Cal

No-Cooking Daily Menu 7

BREAKFAST	Calories	Totals
Orange juice (½ cup)	50	
Wheat Chex (¾ cup) + ½ cup skim milk	200	
Coffee	10	260 Cal
SNACK		
Fresh fruit in season (apple, peach, etc)	70	
Coffee or tea	10	80 Cal
LUNCH		
Soup (Appendix B - page 171)	110	
Whole-grain bread (1 slice)	70	
Coffee or tea	10	190 Cal
SNACK		
Handful unsalted mixed nuts	100	
Coffee or tea	10	110 Cal
DINNER		
Frozen Entrée (Appendix D - page 175)	290	
"Big-Bowl Salad"	150	
Water	0	440 Cal
SNACK		
Popcorn Mini Bag	110	
Coffee or tea	10	120 Cal
		1200 Cal

No-Cooking Daily Menu 8

BREAKFAST	Calories	Totals
Fresh or frozen strawberries (½ cup)	25	
Kashi Go Lean Waffles (2)	150	
Light Syrup (2 Tbsp)	50	
Coffee	10	235 Cal
SNACK		
Yogurt (4 oz, non-fat any flavor)	60	
Coffee or tea	10	70 Cal
LUNCH		
Chicken, Bacon Ranch*	270	
Laughing Cow Light Cheese** (1 wedge)	35	
Fresh fruit in season (apple, plum, etc)	70	
Diet soda or water	0	375 Cal
* Hot Pockets (wrap) or if unavailable an equivalent food.		
** If unavailable an equivalent food.		
SNACK		
Coffee or tea	10	10 Cal
DINNER		
Frozen Entrée (Appendix D - page 175)	270	
"Big-Bowl Salad"	150	
Whole-grain bread (1 slice)	70	
Water with lemon wedge	15	505 Cal
SNACK		
Coffee or tea	10	10 Cal
		1205 Cal

No-Cooking Daily Menu 9

BREAKFAST	Calories	Totals
Grapefruit (½)	75	
Soft-boiled egg	80	
Whole grain toast (1 slice)	70	
Coffee	10	235 Cal
SNACK		
Yogurt (4 oz, non-fat any flavor)	60	
Coffee or tea	10	70 Cal
LUNCH		
Turkey frank (2 oz) with mustard & relish	150	
Hot-dog bun	130	
Diet soda or water	0	280 Cal
SNACK		
Coffee or tea	10	10 Cal
DINNER		
Frozen Entrée (Appendix D - page 175)	320	
"Big-Bowl Salad"	150	
Water with lemon wedge	15	485 Cal
SNACK		
Popcorn Mini Bag	110	
Coffee or tea	10	120 Cal
		1200 Cal

No-Cooking Daily Menu 10

BREAKFAST	Calories	Totals
Fresh sliced orange	75	
Cheerios (1 cup) + ½ cup skim milk + about 15 raisins	190	
Coffee	10	275 Cal
SNACK		
Coffee or tea	10	10 Cal
LUNCH		
Subway 6" (Ham, Cheese + veggies)	260	
Fresh fruit in season (apple, peach, etc)	70	
Diet soda (or water)	0	330 Cal
SNACK		
Handful unsalted mixed nuts	100	
Coffee or tea	10	110 Cal
DINNER		
Frozen Entrée (Appendix D - page 175)	230	
"Big-Bowl Salad"	150	
Whole-grain bread (1 slice)	70	
Water with lemon wedge	15	465 Cal
SNACK		
Coffee or tea	10	10 Cal
		1200 Cal

No-Cooking Daily Menu 11

BREAKFAST	Calories	Totals
Grapefruit (½)	75	
Scrambled egg	80	
Whole-grain toast (1 slice)	70	
Coffee	10	235 Cal
SNACK		
Fresh fruit in season (apple, peach, etc)	70	
Coffee or tea	10	80 Cal
LUNCH		
Soup (Appendix B - page 171)*	240	
Small whole-grain roll	80	
Water	0	320 Cal
SNACK		
Yogurt (4 oz, non-fat any flavor)	60	
Coffee or tea	10	70 Cal
DINNER		
Frozen Entrée (Appendix D - page 175)	320	
"Big-Bowl Salad"	150	
Hot or ice tea	10	480 Cal
SNACK		
Coffee or tea	10	10 Cal
		1195 Cal

No-Cooking Daily Menu 12

BREAKFAST	Calories	Totals
Orange juice (½ cup)	50	
Shredded Wheat (1 cup) + ½ cup skim milk + ½ banana	260	
Coffee	10	320 Cal
SNACK		
Coffee or tea	10	10 Cal
LUNCH		
Peanut butter (2 Tbsp) on 2 slices whole-grain bread	340	
Skim milk (6 oz)	70	410 Cal
SNACK		
Fresh fruit in season (peach, plum, etc)	70	
Coffee or tea	10	80 Cal
DINNER		
Frozen Entrée (Appendix D - page 175)	210	
"Big-Bowl Salad"	150	
Water with lemon wedge	15	375 Cal
SNACK		
Coffee or tea	10	10 Cal
		1205 Cal

No-Cooking Daily Menu 13

BREAKFAST	Calories	Totals
Fresh sliced orange	75	
Wheaties (¾ cup) + ½ cup skim milk + ½ banana	190	
Coffee	10	275 Cal
SNACK		
Fresh fruit in season (apple, peach, etc)	70	
Coffee or tea	10	80 Cal
LUNCH		
Soup (Appendix B - page 171)	130	
Small whole-grain roll	80	
Water	0	210 Cal
SNACK		
Coffee or tea	10	10 Cal
DINNER		
Frozen Entrée (Appendix D - page 175)	310	
"Big-Bowl Salad"	150	
Diet soda (or water)	0	460 Cal
SNACK		
Skinny Cow Ice Cream Sandwich	160	
Coffee or tea	10	170 Cal
		1205 Cal

No-Cooking Daily Menu 14

BREAKFAST	Calories	Totals
Orange juice (½ cup)	50	
Wheat Chex (¾ cup) + ½ cup skim milk + ½ banana	250	
Coffee	10	310 Cal
SNACK		
Yogurt (4 oz, non-fat any flavor)	60	
Coffee or tea	10	70 Cal
LUNCH		
Chicken Pot Pie*	230	
Fresh fruit in season (apple, plum, etc)	70	
Hot or iced tea	10	310 Cal
* Hot Pockets (wrap) or if unavailable an equivalent food.		
SNACK		
Coffee or tea	10	10 Cal
DINNER		
Frozen Entrée (Appendix D - page 175)	230	
"Big-Bowl Salad"	150	
Water with lemon wedge	15	395 Cal
SNACK		
Nature Valley Crunchy Granola bar	95	
Coffee or tea	10	105 Cal
		1200 Cal

No-Cooking Daily Menu 15

BREAKFAST	Calories	Totals
Cantaloupe (½ medium)	50	
Scrambled egg	80	
Toasted raisin bread (1 slice)	75	
Coffee	10	215 Cal
SNACK		
Yogurt (4 oz, non-fat any flavor)	60	
Coffee or tea	10	70 Cal
LUNCH		
Soup (Appendix B - page 171)	170	
String cheese (1 piece, any brand - 80 Cal max)	80	
Fresh fruit in season (apple, plum, etc)	70	
Water	0	320 Cal
SNACK		
Handful unsalted mixed nuts	100	
Coffee or tea	10	110 Cal
DINNER		
Frozen Entrée (Appendix D - page 175)	250	
"Big-Bowl Salad"	150	
Whole-grain bread (1 slice)	70	
Water	0	470 Cal
SNACK		
Coffee or tea	10	10 Cal
		1195 Cal

No-Cooking Daily Menu 16

BREAKFAST	Calories	Totals
Grapefruit (½)	75	
Cheerios (1 cup) + ½ cup skim milk + about 15 raisins	190	
Coffee	10	275 Cal
SNACK		
Coffee or tea	10	10 Cal
LUNCH		
Cottage cheese (1 cup low fat)	180	
Fresh fruit in season (apple, plum, etc)	70	
Small whole-grain roll	80	
Coffee or tea	10	340 Cal
SNACK		
Coffee or tea	10	10 Cal
DINNER		
Frozen Entrée (Appendix D - page 175)	210	
"Big-Bowl Salad"	150	
Whole-grain bread (1 slice)	70	
Water with lemon wedge	15	445 Cal
SNACK		
Popcorn Mini Bag	110	
Coffee or tea	10	120 Cal
		1200 Cal

No-Cooking Daily Menu 17

BREAKFAST	Calories	Totals
Grapefruit (½)	75	
Fried egg	80	
Whole-grain toast (1 slice)	70	
Coffee	10	235 Cal
SNACK		
Yogurt (4 oz, non-fat any flavor)	60	
Coffee or tea	10	70 Cal
LUNCH		
Roast beef (2 oz) sandwich on whole-grain bread	305	
Diet soda or water	0	305 Cal
SNACK		
Coffee or tea	10	10 Cal
DINNER		
Frozen Entrée (Appendix D - page 175)	250	
"Big-Bowl Salad"	150	
Fresh fruit in season (peach, plum, etc)	70	
Water with lemon wedge	15	485 Cal
SNACK		
Graham crackers (3 squares)	90	
Coffee or tea	10	100 Cal
		1205 Cal

No-Cooking Daily Menu 18

BREAKFAST	Calories	Totals
Tomato juice (½ cup)	20	
Shredded Wheat (1 cup) + ½ cup skim milk + ½ banana	260	
Coffee	10	290 Cal
SNACK		
Yogurt (4 oz, non-fat any flavor)	60	
Coffee or tea	10	70 Cal
LUNCH		
Southwest-Style Taco*	270	
Fresh fruit in season (peach, plum, etc)	70	
Diet soda (or water)	0	340 Cal
* Hot Pockets (wrap) or if unavailable an equivalent food.		
SNACK		
Coffee or tea	10	10 Cal
DINNER		
Frozen Entrée (Appendix D - page 175)	260	
"Big-Bowl Salad"	150	
Whole-grain bread (1 slice)	70	
Water	0	480 Cal
SNACK		
Coffee or tea	10	10 Cal
		1200 Cal

No-Cooking Daily Menu 19

BREAKFAST	Calories	Totals
Cantaloupe (½ medium)	50	
Wheat Chex (¾ cup) + ½ cup skim milk + ½ banana	250	
Coffee	10	310 Cal
SNACK		
Fresh fruit in season (apple, plum, etc)	70	
Coffee or tea	10	80 Cal
LUNCH		
Subway 6" (Turkey Breast, Cheese + veggies)	230	
Hot or iced tea	10	240 Cal
SNACK		
Coffee or tea	10	10 Cal
DINNER		
Frozen Entrée (Appendix D - page 175)	230	
"Big-Bowl Salad"	150	
Whole-grain bread (1 slice)	70	
Water	0	440 Cal
SNACK		
Popcorn Mini Bag	110	110 Cal
		1200 Cal

No-Cooking Daily Menu 20

BREAKFAST	Calories	Totals
Fresh or frozen strawberries (½ cup)	25	
Kashi Go Lean Waffles (2)	150	
Light Syrup (2 Tbsp)	50	
Coffee	10	235 Cal
SNACK		
Yogurt (4 oz, non-fat any flavor)	60	
Coffee or tea	10	70 Cal
LUNCH		
Ham (2 oz) with mustard on 2 slices rye bread	300	
Pickle spear	0	
Fresh fruit in season (peach, plum, etc)	70	
Hot or iced tea	10	380 Cal
SNACK		
Nature Valley Crunchy Granola bar	95	
Coffee or tea	10	105 Cal
DINNER		
Frozen Entrée (Appendix D - page 175)	240	
"Big-Bowl Salad"	150	
Hot or iced tea	10	400 Cal
SNACK		
Coffee or tea	10	10 Cal
		1200 Cal

No-Cooking Daily Menu 21

BREAKFAST	Calories	Totals
Orange juice (½ cup)	50	
Soft-boiled egg	80	
Whole-grain toast (1 slice)	70	
Coffee	10	210 Cal
SNACK		
Yogurt (4 oz, non-fat any flavor)	60	
Coffee or tea	10	70 Cal
LUNCH		
Soup (Appendix B - page 171)*	260	
Small whole-grain roll	80	
Coffee or tea	10	350 Cal
* Enjoy 2 servings of a 130 Calorie soup.		
SNACK		
Fresh fruit in season (apple, pear, etc)	70	
Coffee or tea	10	80 Cal
DINNER		
Frozen Entrée (Appendix D - page 175)	260	
"Big-Bowl Salad"	150	
Whole-grain bread (1 slice)	70	
Water	0	480 Cal
SNACK		
Coffee or tea	10	10 Cal
		1200 Cal

No-Cooking Daily Menu 22

BREAKFAST	Calories	Totals
Tomato juice (½ cup)	20	
Cheerios (1 cup) + ½ cup skim milk + about 15 raisins	190	
Coffee	10	220 Cal
SNACK		
Coffee or tea	10	10 Cal
LUNCH		
Cottage cheese (1 cup low fat)	180	
Fresh fruit in season (apple, peach, etc)	70	
Whole-grain bread (1 slice)	70	
Coffee or tea	10	330 Cal
SNACK		
Handful unsalted mixed nuts	100	
Coffee or tea	10	110 Cal
DINNER		
Frozen Entrée (Appendix D - page 175)	290	
"Big-Bowl Salad"	150	
Small whole-grain roll	80	
Water	0	520 Cal
SNACK		
Coffee or tea	10	10 Cal
		1200 Cal

No-Cooking Daily Menu 23

BREAKFAST	Calories	Totals
Cantaloupe (½ medium)	50	
Scrambled egg	80	
Toasted whole-grain bread (1 slice)	70	
Coffee	10	210 Cal
SNACK		
Yogurt (4 oz, non-fat any flavor)	60	
Coffee or tea	10	70 Cal
LUNCH		
Soup (Appendix B - page 171)	140	
Whole-grain bread (1 slice)	70	
Coffee or tea	10	220 Cal
SNACK		
Handful unsalted mixed nuts	100	
Coffee or tea	10	110 Cal
DINNER		
Frozen Entrée (Appendix D - page 175)	250	
"Big-Bowl Salad"	150	
Fresh fruit in season (apple, plum, etc)	70	
Water with lemon wedge	15	485 Cal
SNACK		
Nature Valley Crunchy Granola bar	95	
Coffee or tea	10	105 Cal
		1200 Cal

No-Cooking Daily Menu 24

BREAKFAST	Calories	Totals
Cantaloupe (½ medium)	50	
Oatmeal (½ cup dry) + ½ cup skim milk + 15	220	
Coffee	10	280 Cal
SNACK		
Yogurt (4 oz, non-fat any flavor)	60	
Coffee or tea	10	70 Cal
LUNCH		
Subway 6" (Roast Beef, Cheese + veggies)	245	
Fresh fruit in season (pear, plum, etc)	70	
Diet soda or water	0	315 Cal
SNACK		
Coffee or tea	10	10 Cal
DINNER		
Frozen Entrée (Appendix D - page 175)	280	
"Big-Bowl Salad"	150	
Whole-grain bread (1 slice)	70	
Water with lemon wedge	15	515 Cal
SNACK		
Coffee or tea	10	10 Cal
		1200 Cal

No-Cooking Daily Menu 25

BREAKFAST	Calories	Totals
Orange juice (½ cup)	50	
Wheaties (¾ cup) + ½ cup skim milk + ½ banana	190	
Coffee	10	250 Cal
SNACK		
Fresh fruit in season (peach, plum, etc)	70	
Coffee or tea	10	80 Cal
LUNCH		
Soup (Appendix B - page 171)	170	
Small whole-grain roll	80	
Coffee or tea	10	260 Cal
SNACK		
Coffee or tea	10	10 Cal
DINNER		
Frozen Entrée (Appendix D - page 175)	250	
"Big-Bowl Salad"	150	
Whole-grain bread (1 slice)	70	
Water with lemon wedge	15	485 Cal
SNACK		
Popcorn Mini Bag*	110	
Coffee or tea	10	120 Cal
* Such as Orville Redenbacher's Smart Pop		1205 Cal

No-Cooking Daily Menu 26

BREAKFAST	Calories	Totals
Fresh or frozen strawberries (½ cup)	25	
Kashi Go Lean Waffles (2)	150	
Light Syrup (2 Tbsp)	50	
Coffee	10	235 Cal
SNACK		
Yogurt (4 oz, non-fat any flavor)	60	
Coffee or tea	10	70 Cal
LUNCH		
Chicken Broccoli & Cheese*	270	
Fresh fruit in season (apple, peach, plum, etc)	70	
Diet soda (or water)	0	340 Cal
* Hot Pockets (wrap)		
SNACK		
Handful unsalted mixed nuts	100	
Coffee or tea	10	110 Cal
DINNER		
Frozen Entrée (Appendix D - page 175)	200	
"Big-Bowl Salad"	150	
Whole-grain bread (1 slice)	70	
Water with lemon wedge	15	435 Cal
SNACK		
Coffee or tea	10	10 Cal
		1200 Cal

No-Cooking Daily Menu 27

BREAKFAST	Calories	Totals
Orange juice (½ cup)	50	
Cheerios (1 cup) + ½ cup skim milk + about 15 raisins	190	
Coffee	10	250 Cal
SNACK		
Fresh fruit in season (plum, peach, etc)	70	
Coffee or tea	10	80 Cal
LUNCH		
Subway 6" (Turkey Breast, Cheese + veggies)*	230	
Hot or iced tea	10	240 Cal
SNACK		
Yogurt (4 oz, non-fat any flavor)	60	
Coffee or tea	10	70 Cal
DINNER		
Frozen Entrée (Appendix D - page 175)	330	
"Big-Bowl Salad"	150	
Whole grain bread (1 slice)	70	
Water	0	550 Cal
SNACK		
Coffee or tea	10	10 Cal
		1200 Cal

No-Cooking Daily Menu 28

BREAKFAST	Calories	Totals
Fresh or frozen strawberries (½ cup)	25	
Kashi Go Lean Waffles (2)	150	
Light Syrup (2 Tbsp)	50	
Coffee	10	235 Cal
SNACK		
Yogurt (4 oz, non-fat any flavor)	60	
Coffee or tea	10	70 Cal
LUNCH		
Ham (2 oz) with mustard on 2 slices rye bread	300	
Laughing Cow Light Cheese (1 wedge)	35	
Fresh fruit in season (apple, peach, etc)	70	
Coffee or tea	10	415 Cal
SNACK		
Popcorn Mini Bag	110	
Coffee or tea	10	120 Cal
DINNER		
Frozen Entrée (Appendix D - page 175)	180	
"Big-Bowl Salad"	150	
Water with lemon wedge	15	345 Cal
SNACK		
Coffee or tea	10	10 Cal
		1195 Cal

No-Cooking Daily Menu 29

BREAKFAST	Calories	Totals
Grapefruit (½)	75	
Fried egg	80	
Turkey bacon (1 slice)	35	
Whole grain toast (1 slice)	70	
Coffee	10	270 Cal
SNACK		
Coffee or tea	10	10 Cal
LUNCH		
Salad (3 oz canned tuna, 1 tsp Evoo, onions, celery)	175	
Rye bread (1 slice)	70	
Small bunch of grapes	65	
Hot or iced tea	10	320 Cal
SNACK		
Handful unsalted mixed nuts	100	
Coffee or tea	10	110 Cal
DINNER		
Frozen Entrée (Appendix D - page 175)	260	
"Big-Bowl Salad"	150	
Whole-grain bread (1 slice)	70	
Water	0	480 Cal
SNACK		
Coffee or tea	10	10 Cal
		1200 Cal

No-Cooking Daily Menu 30

BREAKFAST	Calories	Totals
Grapefruit (½)	75	
Wheaties (¾ cup) + ½ cup skim milk + ½ banana	190	
Coffee	10	275 Cal
SNACK		
Coffee or tea	10	10 Cal
LUNCH		
Cottage cheese (1 cup low fat)	180	
Fresh fruit in season (peach, plum, etc)	70	
Small whole-grain roll	80	
Diet soda or water	0	330 Cal
SNACK		
Coffee or tea	10	10 Cal
DINNER		
Frozen Entrée (Appendix D - page 175)	270	
"Big-Bowl Salad"	150	
Whole-grain bread (1 slice)	70	
Diet soda (or water)	0	485 Cal
SNACK		
Fiber One Chocolate Fudge Brownie	90	90 Cal
		1200 Cal

BREAKFAST	Calories	Totals
Cantaloupe (½ medium)	50	
Scrambled egg	80	
Toasted raisin bread (1 slice)	75	
Coffee	10	215 Cal
SNACK		
Yogurt (4 oz, non-fat any flavor)	60	
Coffee or tea	10	70 Cal
LUNCH		
Soup (Appendix B - page 171)*	280	
Small whole-grain roll	80	
Water with lemon wedge	15	375 Cal
* Enjoy 2 servings of a 140 Calorie soup.		
SNACK		
Fresh fruit in season (pear, plum, etc)	70	
Coffee or tea	10	80 Cal
DINNER		
Frozen Entrée (Appendix D - page 175)	210	
"Big-Bowl Salad"	150	
Small whole-grain roll	80	
Water with lemon wedge	15	455 Cal
SNACK		
Coffee or tea	10	10 Cal
		1205 Cal

No-Cooking Daily Menu 32

BREAKFAST	Calories	Totals
Tomato juice (½ cup)	20	
Shredded Wheat (1 cup) + ½ cup skim milk + ½ banana	265	
Coffee	10	295 Cal
SNACK		
Yogurt (4 oz, non-fat any flavor)	60	
Coffee or tea	10	70 Cal
LUNCH		
Southwest-Style Taco*	270	
Fresh fruit in season (pear, peach, etc)	70	
Diet soda or water	0	340 Cal
* Hot Pockets (wrap)		
SNACK		
Coffee or tea	10	10 Cal
DINNER		
Frozen Entrée (Appendix D - page 175)	210	
"Big-Bowl Salad"	150	
Fresh blueberries, cherries or grapes (1 cup)	100	
Water with lemon wedge	15	475 Cal
SNACK		
Coffee or tea	10	10 Cal
		1200 Cal

No-Cooking Daily Menu 33

BREAKFAST	Calories	Totals
Orange juice (½ cup)	50	
Wheat Chex (¾ cup) + ½ cup skim milk + ½ banana	250	
Coffee	10	310 Cal
SNACK		
Fresh fruit in season (apple, peach, etc)	70	
Coffee or tea	10	80 Cal
LUNCH		
Soup (Appendix B - page 171)	90	
String cheese (1 piece, any brand)	80	
Whole-grain bread (1 slice)	70	
Coffee or tea	10	250 Cal
SNACK		
Coffee or tea	10	10 Cal
DINNER		
Frozen Entrée (Appendix D - page 175)	320	
"Big-Bowl Salad"	150	
Whole-grain bread (1 slice)	70	
Water	0	540 Cal
SNACK		
Coffee or tea	10	10 Cal
		1200 Cal

No-Cooking Daily Menu 34

BREAKFAST	Calories	Totals
Orange juice (½ cup)	50	
Kashi Go Lean Waffles (2)	150	
Light Syrup (2 Tbsp)	50	
Coffee	10	260 Cal
SNACK		
Yogurt (4 oz, non-fat any flavor)	60	
Coffee or tea	10	70 Cal
LUNCH		
Chicken, Bacon Ranch*	270	
Fresh fruit in season (apple, peach, etc)	70	
Hot or iced tea	10	350 Cal
* Hot Pockets (wrap)		
SNACK		
Coffee or tea	10	10 Cal
DINNER		
Frozen Entrée (Appendix D - page 175)	270	
"Big-Bowl Salad"	150	
Whole-grain bread (1 slice)	70	
Water with lemon wedge	15	505 Cal
SNACK		
Coffee or tea	10	10 Cal
		1205 Cal

No-Cooking Daily Menu 35

BREAKFAST	Calories	Totals
Grapefruit (½)	75	
Fried egg	80	
Whole-grain toast (1 slice)	70	
Coffee	10	235 Cal
SNACK		
Yogurt (4 oz, non-fat any flavor)	60	
Coffee or tea	10	70 Cal
LUNCH		
Subway 6" Sandwich (Roast Beef, Cheese + veggies)	245	
Fresh fruit in season (pear, plum, etc)	70	
Hot or iced tea	10	325 Cal
SNACK		
Coffee or tea	10	10 Cal
DINNER		
Frozen Entrée (Appendix D - page 175)	310	
"Big-Bowl Salad"	150	
Fresh fruit in season (apple, plum, etc)	70	
Water with lemon wedge	15	545 Cal
SNACK		
Coffee or tea	10	10 Cal
		1195 Cal

No-Cooking Daily Menu 36

BREAKFAST	Calories	Totals
Fresh sliced orange	75	
Cheerios (1 cup) + ½ cup skim milk + about 15 raisins	190	
Coffee	10	275 Cal
SNACK		
Coffee or tea	10	10 Cal
LUNCH		
Cottage cheese (1 cup low fat)	180	
Fresh fruit in season (peach, plum, etc)	70	
Small whole-grain roll	80	
Coffee or tea	10	340 Cal
SNACK		
Coffee or tea	10	10 Cal
DINNER		
Frozen Entrée (Appendix D - page 175)	220	
"Big-Bowl Salad"	150	
Whole-grain bread (1 slice)	70	
Water	0	440 Cal
SNACK		
Popcorn Mini Bag	110	
Coffee or tea	10	120 Cal
		1195 Cal

No-Cooking Daily Menu 37

BREAKFAST	Calories	Totals
Grapefruit (½)	75	
Soft-boiled egg	80	
Whole-grain toast (1 slice)	70	
Coffee	10	235 Cal
SNACK		
Fresh fruit in season (peach, plum, etc)	70	
Coffee or tea	10	80 Cal
LUNCH		
Salad (3 oz canned tuna, 1 tsp Evoo, onions, celery)	175	
Whole-grain bread (1 slice)	70	
Fresh fruit in season (peach, plum, etc)	70	
Diet soda or water	0	315 Cal
SNACK		
Yogurt (4 oz, non-fat any flavor)	60	
Coffee or tea	10	70 Cal
DINNER		
Frozen Entrée (Appendix D - page 175)	330	
"Big-Bowl Salad"	150	
Water with lemon wedge	15	495 Cal
SNACK		
Coffee or tea	10	10 Cal
		1195 Cal

No-Cooking Daily Menu 38

BREAKFAST	Calories	Totals
Orange juice (½ cup)	50	
Shredded Wheat (1 cup) + ½ cup skim milk + ½ banana	260	
Coffee	10	320 Cal
SNACK		
Fresh fruit in season (pear, plum, etc)	70	
Coffee or tea	10	80 Cal
LUNCH		
Peanut butter (2 Tbsp) on 2 slices whole-grain bread	340	
Skim milk (6 oz)	70	
Water	0	410 Cal
SNACK		
Coffee or tea	10	10 Cal
DINNER		
Frozen Entrée (Appendix D - page 175)	210	
"Big-Bowl Salad"	150	
Water with lemon wedge	15	355 Cal
SNACK		
Coffee or tea	10	10 Cal
		1205 Cal

No-Cooking Daily Menu 39

BREAKFAST	Calories	Totals
Fresh sliced orange	75	
Wheaties (¾ cup) + ½ cup skim milk + ½ banana	190	
Coffee	10	275 Cal
SNACK		
Fresh fruit in season (apple, plum, etc)	70	
Coffee or tea	10	80 Cal
LUNCH		
Soup (Appendix B - page 171)	100	
Small whole-grain roll	80	
Coffee or tea	10	190 Cal
SNACK		
Coffee or tea	10	10 Cal
DINNER		
Frozen Entrée (Appendix D - page 175)	330	
"Big-Bowl Salad"	150	
Water with lemon wedge	15	495 Cal
SNACK		
Kashi Chewy Granola Bar	140	
Coffee or tea	10	150 Cal
		1200 Cal

No-Cooking Daily Menu 40

BREAKFAST	Calories	Totals
Orange juice (½ cup)	50	
Wheat Chex (¾ cup) + ½ cup skim milk + ½ banana	250	
Coffee	10	310 Cal
SNACK		
Yogurt (4 oz, non-fat any flavor)	60	
Coffee or tea	10	70 Cal
LUNCH		
Turkey frank (2 oz) with mustard & relish	150	
Hot-dog bun	130	
Hot or iced tea	10	290 Cal
SNACK		
Coffee or tea	10	10 Cal
DINNER		
Frozen Entrée (Appendix D - page 175)	220	
"Big-Bowl Salad"	150	
Whole-grain bread (1 slice)	70	
Water	0	440 Cal
SNACK		
Coffee or tea	10	10 Cal
		1200 Cal

BREAKFAST	Calories	Totals
Cantaloupe (½ medium)	50	
Fried egg	80	
Toasted raisin bread (1 slice)	75	
Coffee	10	215 Cal
SNACK		
Yogurt (4 oz, non-fat any flavor)	60	
Coffee or tea	10	70 Cal
LUNCH		
Soup (Appendix B - page 171)*	170	
String cheese (1 piece, any brand)	80	
Coffee or tea	10	260 Cal
SNACK		
Coffee or tea	10	10 Cal
DINNER		
Frozen Entrée (Appendix D - page 175)	250	
"Big-Bowl Salad"	150	
Whole-grain bread (1 slice)	70	
Fresh fruit in season (peach, plum, etc)	70	
Water with lemon wedge	15	555 Cal
SNACK		
Nature Valley Crunchy Granola bar	95	95 Cal
		1205 Cal

No-Cooking Daily Menu 42

BREAKFAST	Calories	Totals
Grapefruit (½)	75	
Cheerios (1 cup) + ½ cup skim milk + about 15 raisins	190	
Coffee	10	275 Cal
SNACK		
Coffee or tea	10	10 Cal
LUNCH		
Cottage cheese (1 cup low fat)	180	
Fresh fruit in season (plum, peach, etc)	70	
Small whole-grain roll	80	
Coffee or tea	10	340 Cal
SNACK		
Coffee or tea	10	10 Cal
DINNER		
Frozen Entrée (Appendix D - page 175)	230	
"Big-Bowl Salad"	150	
Whole-grain bread (1 slice)	70	
Water	0	450 Cal
SNACK		
Popcorn Mini Bag	110	
Coffee or tea	10	120 Cal
		1205 Cal

No-Cooking Daily Menu 43

BREAKFAST	Calories	Totals
Grapefruit (½)	75	
Scrambled egg	80	
Whole grain toast (1 slice)	70	
Coffee	10	235 Cal
SNACK		
Yogurt (4 oz, non-fat any flavor)	60	
Coffee or tea	10	70 Cal
LUNCH		
Subway 6" Sandwich (Turkey Breast, Cheese + veggies)	230	
Diet soda (or water)	0	230 Cal
SNACK		
Coffee or tea	10	10 Cal
DINNER		
Frozen Entrée (Appendix D - page 175)	270	
"Big-Bowl Salad"	150	
Whole-grain bread (1 slice)	70	
Water	0	490 Cal
SNACK		
Fresh fruit in season (apple, plum, etc)	70	
Coffee or tea	10	80 Cal
		1195 Cal

No-Cooking Daily Menu 44

BREAKFAST	Calories	Totals
Tomato juice (½ cup)	20	
Shredded Wheat (1 cup) + ½ cup skim milk + ½ banana	260	
Coffee	10	290 Cal
SNACK		
Yogurt (4 oz, non-fat any flavor)	60	
Coffee or tea	10	70 Cal
LUNCH		
Frozen Entrée (Go to **Appendix D** - page 175)	280	
Fresh fruit in season (apple, peach, etc)	70	
Diet soda (or water)	0	350 Cal
SNACK		
Coffee or tea	10	10 Cal
DINNER		
Frozen Entrée (Appendix D - page 175)	250	
"Big-Bowl Salad"	150	
Whole-grain bread (1 slice)	70	
Water	0	480 Cal
SNACK		
Coffee or tea	10	10 Cal
		1200 Cal

No-Cooking Daily Menu 45

BREAKFAST	Calories	Totals
Cantaloupe (½ medium)	50	
Wheat Chex (¾ cup) + ½ cup skim milk + ½ banana	250	
Coffee	10	310 Cal
SNACK		
Coffee or tea	10	10 Cal
LUNCH		
Soup (Appendix B - page 171)	120	
Whole-grain bread (1 slice)	70	
Coffee or tea	10	200 Cal
SNACK		
Fresh fruit in season (peach, plum, etc)	70	
Coffee or tea	10	80 Cal
DINNER		
Frozen Entrée (Appendix D - page 175)	270	
"Big-Bowl Salad"	150	
Whole-grain bread (1 slice)	70	
Water	0	490 Cal
SNACK		
Handful unsalted mixed nuts	100	
Coffee or tea	10	110 Cal
		1200 Cal

No-Cooking Daily Menu 46

BREAKFAST	Calories	Totals
Orange juice (½ cup)	50	
Wheat Chex (¾ cup) + ½ cup skim milk + ½ banana	250	
Coffee	10	310 Cal
SNACK		
Coffee or tea	10	10 Cal
LUNCH		
Chicken Pot Pie*	230	
Fresh fruit in season (peach, plum, etc)	70	
Coffee or tea	10	310 Cal
* Hot Pockets (wrap)		
SNACK		
Coffee or tea	10	10 Cal
DINNER		
Frozen Entrée (Appendix D - page 175)	220	
"Big-Bowl Salad"	150	
Whole-grain bread (1 slice)	70	
Water	0	450 Cal
SNACK		
Handful unsalted mixed nuts	100	
Coffee or tea	10	110 Cal
		1200 Cal

No-Cooking Daily Menu 47

BREAKFAST	Calories	Totals
Cantaloupe (½ medium)	50	
Scrambled egg	80	
Toasted raisin bread (1 slice)	75	
Coffee	10	215 Cal
SNACK		
Yogurt (4 oz, non-fat, any flavor)	60	
Coffee or tea	10	70 Cal
LUNCH		
Soup (Appendix B - page 171)	160	
Fresh fruit in season (plum, pear, etc)	70	
Coffee or tea	10	240 Cal
SNACK		
Handful unsalted mixed nuts	100	
Coffee or tea	10	110 Cal
DINNER		
Frozen Entrée (Appendix D - page 175)	290	
"Big-Bowl Salad"	150	
Water	0	440 Cal
SNACK		
Popcorn Mini Bag	110	
Coffee or tea	10	120 Cal
		1195 Cal

No-Cooking Daily Menu 48

BREAKFAST	Calories	Totals
Grapefruit (½)	75	
Cheerios (1 cup) + ½ cup skim milk + about 15 raisins	190	
Coffee	10	275 Cal
SNACK		
Coffee or tea	10	10 Cal
LUNCH		
Subway 6" (Ham, Cheese + veggies)	260	
Fresh fruit in season (apple, plum, etc)	70	
Hot or iced tea	10	340 Cal
SNACK		
Coffee or tea	10	10 Cal
DINNER		
Frozen Entrée (Appendix D - page 175)	220	
"Big-Bowl Salad"	150	
Whole-grain bread (1 slice)	70	
Water with lemon wedge	15	455 Cal
SNACK		
Handful unsalted mixed nuts	100	
Coffee or tea	10	110 Cal
		1200 Cal

No-Cooking Daily Menu 49

BREAKFAST	Calories	Totals
Grapefruit (½)	75	
Fried egg	80	
Whole grain toast (1 slice)	70	
Coffee	10	235 Cal
SNACK		
Yogurt (4 oz, non-fat, any flavor)	60	
Coffee or tea	10	70 Cal
LUNCH		
Soup (Appendix B - page 171)*	240	
Small whole-grain roll	80	
Coffee or tea	10	330 Cal
SNACK		
Coffee or tea	10	10 Cal
DINNER		
Frozen Entrée (Appendix D - page 175)	320	
"Big-Bowl Salad"	150	
Fresh fruit in season (peach, plum, etc)	70	
Hot or iced tea	10	550 Cal
SNACK		
Coffee or tea	10	10 Cal
		1205 Cal

No-Cooking Daily Menu 50

BREAKFAST	Calories	Totals
Tomato juice (½ cup)	20	
Shredded Wheat (1 cup) + ½ cup skim milk + ½ banana	260	
Coffee	10	290 Cal
SNACK		
Yogurt (4 oz, non-fat, any flavor)	60	
Coffee or tea	10	70 Cal
LUNCH		
Salad (3 oz canned tuna, 1 tsp Evoo, onions, celery)	175	
Rye bread (1 slice)	70	
Small bunch of grapes	65	
Hot or iced tea	10	320 Cal
SNACK		
Coffee or tea	10	10 Cal
DINNER		
Frozen Entrée (Appendix D - page 175)	280	
"Big-Bowl Salad"	150	
Whole-grain bread (1 slice)	70	
Water	0	500 Cal
SNACK		
Coffee or tea	10	10 Cal
		1200 Cal

COOKING
Daily Meal Plans

Cooking Daily Menu 1

BREAKFAST	Calories	Totals
Grapefruit (½)	75	
Scrambled egg (See Notes - page 10)	80	
Whole grain toast (1 slice) (See page 10)	70	
Coffee (See page 10)	10	235 Cal
SNACK		
Coffee or tea	10	10 Cal
LUNCH		
Ham (2 oz) with mustard on 2 slices rye bread	290	
Pickle spear	0	
Hot or iced tea	10	300 Cal
SNACK		
Fresh fruit in season (apple, peach, etc)	70	
Coffee or tea	10	80 Cal
DINNER		
Chicken with Peppers & Onions (Recipe 1 page 115)	250	
Sautéed red peppers with onions (Recipe 1)	70	
Green beans (steamed) & mashed cauliflower	25	
Large tossed salad - 1½ Tbsp dressing (See pages 9 & 10)	85	
Water with lemon wedge	15	475 Cal
SNACK		
Graham crackers (2 squares)	60	
Skim milk (4 oz = ½ cup)	45	105 Cal
		1205 Cal

Cooking Daily Menu 2

BREAKFAST	Calories	Totals
Orange juice (½ cup)	50	
Wheaties (¾ cup) + ½ cup skim milk + ½ banana	190	
Coffee	10	250 Cal
SNACK		
Fresh fruit in season (apple, pear, etc)	70	
Coffee or tea	10	80 Cal
LUNCH		
Subway 6" (Turkey Breast, Cheese + veggies)*	230	
Coffee or tea	10	240 Cal
* On half of 9-grain wheat roll.		
SNACK		
Coffee or tea	10	10 Cal
DINNER		
Baked Herb-Crusted Cod (Recipe 2 - page 116)	230	
Spinach (½ cup) steamed with garlic & drizzled	100	
Asparagus (8 spear cooked & drained)	25	
Baked potato (medium size) (No Butter!)	100	
Whole grain bread (1 slice)	70	
Water	0	525 Cal
SNACK		
Fiber One Chocolate Fudge Brownie	90	
Coffee or tea	10	100 Cal
		1205 Cal

Cooking Daily Menu 3

BREAKFAST	Calories	Totals
Fresh or frozen strawberries (½ cup)	25	
French toasted English Muffin (Recipe 3 - page 117)	270	
Light syrup (1 Tbsp)	30	
Coffee	10	335 Cal
SNACK		
Coffee or tea	10	10 Cal
LUNCH		
Salad (3 oz can tuna, 1 tsp Evoo, onions, celery)	175	
Rye bread (1 slice)	70	
Small bunch of grapes	65	
Diet soda or water	0	310 Cal
SNACK		
Coffee or tea	10	10 Cal
DINNER		
Broiled veal chop (4 oz lean)	200	
Corn on the cob (1 medium ear) (No Butter!)	100	
Broccoli (½ cup steamed & drizzled with 1 tsp	70	
Large tossed salad - 1½ Tbsp dressing (See pages 9 &10)	85	
Fresh fruit in season (apple, peach, etc)	70	
Water	0	525 Cal
SNACK		
Coffee or tea	10	10 Cal
		1200 Cal

Cooking Daily Menu 4

BREAKFAST	Calories	Totals
Grapefruit (½)	75	
Cheerios (1 cup) + ½ cup skim milk + about 15 raisins*	190	
Coffee	10	275 Cal
SNACK		
Coffee or tea	10	10 Cal
LUNCH		
Cottage cheese (1 cup low fat)	180	
Large tossed salad with 1½ Tbsp low-cal dressing	70	
Small whole-grain roll	80	
Water	0	330 Cal
SNACK		
Fresh fruit in season (peach, plum, etc)	70	
Coffee or tea	10	80 Cal
DINNER		
Meat Loaf (Recipe 4 - page 118)	290	
One-half acorn squash (baked with ½ tsp maple syrup)	60	
Spinach (½ cup steamed & drizzled with 1 tsp Evoo)	85	
Romaine lettuce, tomato slices, & 1 Tbsp **low-**cal dressing	45	
Water	0	495 Cal
SNACK		
Coffee or tea	10	10 Cal
* See Notes - page 10 re substituting blueberries for raisins		**1200 Cal**

Cooking Daily Menu 5

BREAKFAST	Calories	Totals
Fresh orange sliced	75	
Kashi GoLean cereal (1 cup) + ½ cup skim milk	185	
Coffee	10	270 Cal
SNACK		
Coffee or tea	10	10 Cal
LUNCH		
Soup (Appendix B - page 171)	130	
Whole-grain bread (1 slice)	70	
Raw zucchini slices, celery & carrot sticks	20	
Hot or iced tea	10	230 Cal
SNACK		
Coffee or tea	10	10 Cal
DINNER		
Veal w Mushrooms & Tomato (Recipe 5 - page 119)	520	
Small whole-grain roll	80	
Water	0	600 Cal
SNACK		
Fresh fruit in season (apple, plum, etc)	70	
Coffee or tea	10	80 Cal
		1200 Cal

Cooking Daily Menu 6

BREAKFAST	Calories	Totals
Tomato juice (½ cup)	20	
Shredded Wheat (1 cup) + ½ cup skim milk + ½ banana	265	
Coffee	10	295 Cal
SNACK		
Coffee or tea	10	10 Cal
LUNCH		
Leftover meat loaf (½ Recipe 4) with ketchup	155	
Small whole-grain roll	80	
Lettuce	0	
Fresh or frozen berries (½ cup)	50	
Water	0	285 Cal
SNACK		
Coffee or tea	10	10 Cal
DINNER		
Pizza (Recipe 6 - page 120)	350	
Large tossed salad with 1½ Tbsp low-cal dressing	85	
Fresh fruit in season (apple, plum, etc)	70	
Water	0	550 Cal
SNACK		
Yogurt (4 oz, non-fat any flavor)*	60	
* Such as Dannon Lite & Fit. (Buy 32 oz container & use 6 oz.)		1200 Cal

Cooking Daily Menu 7

BREAKFAST	Calories	Totals
Cantaloupe (½ medium)	50	
Wheaties (¾ cup) + ½ cup skim milk + ½ banana	190	
Coffee	10	250 Cal
SNACK		
Fresh fruit in season (peach, plum, etc)	70	
Coffee or tea	10	80 Cal
LUNCH		
Soup (Appendix B - page 171)	140	
Turkey (1 oz) on 1 slice of rye bread (½ sandwich)	120	
Lettuce & tomato slices	20	
Hot or iced tea	10	290 Cal
SNACK		
Coffee or tea	10	10 Cal
DINNER		
Baked salmon with salsa (Recipe 7 - page 121)	215	
Baked summer squash and zucchini	40	
Brown rice (½ cup – after cooking)	100	
Large tossed salad with 1½ Tbsp low-cal dressing	85	
Water with lemon wedge	15	455 Cal
SNACK		
Popcorn Mini Bag*	110	
Coffee or tea	10	120 Cal
* Such as Orville Redenbacher's Smart Pop		1205 Cal

Cooking Daily Menu 8

BREAKFAST	Calories	Totals
Orange juice (½ cup)	50	
Perfect egg (Recipe 8a - page 122)	80	
Whole-grain toast (1 slice)	70	
Coffee	10	210 Cal
SNACK		
Yogurt (4 oz, non-fat, any flavor)	60	
Coffee or tea	10	70 Cal
LUNCH		
Soup (Appendix B - page 171)	170	
Lettuce & tomato wedges + rye bread (1 slice)	60	
Coffee or tea	10	270 Cal
SNACK		
Handful unsalted mixed nuts	100	
Coffee or tea	10	110 Cal
DINNER		
Veggie burger – (1 patty) (Recipe 8b - page 123)	100	
Low-fat cheddar cheese (1 thin slice)	50	
Seeded hamburger roll	140	
Beets (3 small, boiled, skinned & sliced)	45	
Fresh fruit in season (apple, peach, etc)	70	
Water with lemon wedge	15	420 Cal
SNACK		
100-Calorie Pack Cookies*	100	
Coffee or tea	10	110 Cal
* Such as Nabisco Oreo/Chips Ahoy/etc		1190 Cal

Cooking Daily Menu 9

BREAKFAST	Calories	Totals
Orange juice (½ cup)	50	
Wild blueberry pancakes (Recipe 9 - page 123)	190	
Light syrup (1½ Tbsp)	45	
Coffee	10	295 Cal
SNACK		
Coffee or tea	10	10 Cal
LUNCH		
Peanut butter (2 Tbsp) on 2 slices of whole-grain bread	340	
Skim milk (6 oz)	65	
Fresh fruit in season (apple, plum, etc)	70	475 Cal
SNACK		
Coffee or tea	10	10 Cal
DINNER		
Broiled pork chop (about 4 oz of meat - fat trimmed)	260	
Green peas (½ cup)	55	
Tomato & cucumber salad with 1½ Tbsp low-cal	70	
Water with lemon wedge	15	400 Cal
SNACK		
Coffee or tea	10	10 Cal
		1200 Cal

Cooking Daily Menu 10

BREAKFAST	Calories	Totals
Fresh sliced orange	75	
Cheerios (1 cup) + ½ cup skim milk + about 15 raisins	190	
Coffee	10	275 Cal
SNACK		
Coffee or tea	10	10 Cal
LUNCH		
Subway 6" Sandwich (Ham, Cheese + veggies)*	260	
Fresh fruit in season (apple, peach, etc)	70	
Diet soda (or water)	0	330 Cal
SNACK		
Fresh fruit in season (apple, plum, etc)	70	
Coffee or tea	10	80 Cal
DINNER		
Grilled chicken sausage (2 links about 2½ oz per link)	180	
Artichoke-bean salad (Recipe 10 - page 125)	190	
Green beans (¼ lb – steamed)	25	
Whole-grain bread (1 slice)	70	
Water	0	465 Cal
SNACK		
Coffee or tea	10	10 Cal
		1195 Cal

Cooking Daily Menu 11

BREAKFAST	Calories	Totals
Orange juice (½ cup)	50	
Shredded Wheat (1 cup) + ½ cup skim milk + ½ banana	260	
Coffee	10	320 Cal
SNACK		
Handful unsalted mixed nuts	100	
Coffee or tea	10	110 Cal
LUNCH		
Turkey frank (2 oz) with mustard & relish	150	
Hot-dog bun	130	
Hot or iced tea	10	290 Cal
SNACK		
Coffee or tea	10	10 Cal
DINNER		
Pasta with Marinara sauce (Recipe 11 - page 126)	225	
Large tossed salad with 1½ Tbsp low-cal dressing	85	
Fresh fruit in season (peach, plum, etc)	70	
Italian or French bread (1 slice)	80	
Water	0	460 Cal
SNACK		
Coffee or tea	10	10 Cal
		1200 Cal

Cooking Daily Menu 12

BREAKFAST	Calories	Totals
Fresh or frozen strawberries (1 cup)	**50**	
French toasted English Muffin (Recipe 3 - page 116)	**270**	
Light syrup (1 Tbsp)	**30**	
Coffee	**10**	**360 Cal**
SNACK		
Yogurt (4 oz nonfat, any flavor)	**60**	
Coffee or tea	**10**	**70 Cal**
LUNCH		
Salad (3 oz canned tuna, 1 tsp Evoo, onions, celery)	**175**	
Rye bread (1 slice)	**70**	
Coffee or tea	**10**	**255 Cal**
SNACK		
Coffee or tea	**10**	**10 Cal**
DINNER		
London broil (Recipe 12 - page 127)	**320**	
Brown rice (½ cup – after cooking)	**100**	
Steamed broccoli (1 cup – after cooking)	**50**	
Water with lemon wedge	**15**	**485 Cal**
SNACK		
Coffee or tea	**10**	**10 Cal**
		1190 Cal

Cooking Daily Menu 13

BREAKFAST	Calories	Totals
Orange juice (½ cup)	50	
Kashi GoLean (1 cup) + ½ cup skim milk + ½ banana	235	
Coffee	10	295 Cal
SNACK		
Fresh fruit in season (apple, plum, etc)	70	
Coffee or tea	10	80 Cal
LUNCH		
Soup (Appendix B - page 171)	100	
Small whole-grain roll	80	
Lettuce & sliced tomato with 1 Tbsp low-cal dressing	45	
Hot or iced tea	10	235 Cal
SNACK		
Coffee or tea	10	10 Cal
DINNER		
Baked red snapper (Recipe 13 - page 128)	215	
Wild rice mix (Recipe 13)	160	
Green beans & tomato	75	
Water with lemon wedge	15	465 Cal
SNACK		
Popcorn Mini Bag	110	
Coffee or tea	10	120 Cal
		1205 Cal

Cooking Daily Menu 14

BREAKFAST	Calories	Totals
Cantaloupe (½ medium)	50	
Perfect egg (Recipe 8a - page 122)	80	
Toasted raisin bread (1 slice)	75	
Coffee	10	215 Cal
SNACK		
Yogurt (4 oz, non-fat any flavor)	60	
Coffee or tea	10	70 Cal
LUNCH		
Soup (Appendix B - page 171)	190	
Lettuce & tomato sandwich (Tbsp light mayo)	170	
Cucumber slices and carrots & celery sticks	15	
Hot or iced tea	10	385 Cal
SNACK		
Handful unsalted mixed nuts	100	
Coffee or tea	10	110 Cal
DINNER		
Cajun chicken salad (Recipe 14 - page 129)	330	
Small whole-grain roll	80	
Water with lemon wedge	15	420 Cal
SNACK		
Coffee or tea	10	10 Cal
		1210 Cal

Cooking Daily Menu 15

BREAKFAST	Calories	Totals
Grapefruit (½)	75	
Cheerios (1 cup) + ½ cup skim milk + about 15 raisins	190	
Coffee	10	275 Cal
SNACK		
Coffee or tea	10	10 Cal
LUNCH		
Cottage cheese (1 cup low fat)	180	
Large tossed salad with 1½ Tbsp low-cal dressing	70	
Small whole-grain roll	80	
Hot or iced tea	10	340 Cal
SNACK		
Handful unsalted mixed nuts	100	
Coffee or tea	10	110 Cal
DINNER		
Grilled swordfish (Recipe 15 - page 130)	250	
Grilled potatoes (Recipe 15)	100	
Grilled cherry tomatoes (Recipe 15)	45	
Spinach (½ cup) steamed with garlic & drizzled Evoo	50	
Water with lemon wedge	15	455 Cal
SNACK		
Coffee or tea	10	10 Cal
		1205 Cal

Cooking Daily Menu 16

BREAKFAST	Calories	Totals
Tomato juice (½ cup)	20	
Shredded Wheat (1 cup) + ½ cup skim milk + ½ banana	260	
Coffee	10	290 Cal
SNACK		
Coffee or tea	10	10 Cal
LUNCH		
Ham (2 oz) with mustard on 2 slices rye bread	290	
Pickle spear	0	
Hot or iced tea	10	300 Cal
SNACK		
Yogurt (4 oz, non-fat any flavor)	60	
Coffee or tea	10	70 Cal
DINNER		
Spaghetti alla Puttanesca (Recipe 16 - page 131)	345	
Large tossed salad with 1½ Tbsp low-cal dressing	85	
Italian or French bread (1 slice)	80	
Water	0	510 Cal
SNACK		
Coffee or tea	10	10 Cal
		1190 Cal

Cooking Daily Menu 17

BREAKFAST	Calories	Totals
Fresh or frozen strawberries (1 cup)	25	
French toasted English Muffin (Recipe 3 - page 117)	270	
Light syrup (1 Tbsp)	30	
Coffee	10	335 Cal
SNACK		
Coffee or tea	10	10 Cal
LUNCH		
Soup (Appendix B - page 171)	110	
BLT sandwich (2 slices turkey bacon, 1 Tbsp light	245	
Pickle spear	0	
Hot or iced tea	10	365 Cal
SNACK		
Coffee or tea	10	10 Cal
DINNER		
Shrimp & spinach salad (Recipe 17 - page 132)	310	
Whole-grain bread (1 slice)	70	
Fresh fruit in season (apple, peach, etc)	70	
Water with lemon wedge	15	465 Cal
SNACK		
Coffee or tea	10	10 Cal
		1195 Cal

Cooking Daily Menu 18

BREAKFAST	Calories	Totals
Grapefruit (½)	75	
Cheerios (1 cup) + ½ cup skim milk + about 15 raisins	190	
Coffee	10	275 Cal
SNACK		
Coffee or tea	10	10 Cal
LUNCH		
Subway 6" Sandwich (Roast Beef, Cheese + veggies)*	245	
Diet soda (or water)	0	245 Cal
SNACK		
Coffee or tea	10	10 Cal
DINNER		
Hanger steak (Recipe 18 - page 133)	320	
Roasted potatoes (Recipe 18)	120	
Cherry tomatoes (Recipe 18)	20	
Steamed spinach (½ cup)	25	
Whole-grain bread (1 slice)	70	
Water	0	555 Cal
SNACK		
Coffee or tea	10	10 Cal
		1200 Cal

Cooking Daily Menu 19

BREAKFAST	Calories	Totals
Fresh orange sliced	75	
Soft-boiled egg	80	
Whole-grain toast (1 slice)	70	
Coffee	10	235 Cal
SNACK		
Yogurt (4 oz, non-fat any flavor)	60	
Coffee or tea	10	70 Cal
LUNCH		
Salad - 3 oz canned salmon, 1 tsp Evoo, onions & celery	200	
Lettuce & tomato wedges	20	
Rye bread (1 slice)	70	
Water with lemon wedge	15	305 Cal
SNACK		
Fresh fruit in season (peach, plum, etc)	70	
Coffee or tea	10	80 Cal
DINNER		
Chicken breast (5 oz - broiled)	250	
Four bean plus salad (½ cup) (Recipe 19 - page 134)	135	
Large tossed salad with 1½ Tbsp low-cal dressing	85	
Water with lemon wedge	15	485 Cal
SNACK		
Coffee or tea	10	10 Cal
		1185 Cal

Cooking Daily Menu 20

BREAKFAST	Calories	Totals
Cantaloupe (½ medium)	50	
Wheaties (¾ cup) + ½ cup skim milk + ½ banana	190	
Coffee	10	250 Cal
SNACK		
Handful unsalted mixed nuts	100	
Coffee or tea	10	110 Cal
LUNCH		
Ham (2 oz) with mustard on 2 slices rye bread	300	
Pickle spear	0	
Hot or iced tea	10	315 Cal
SNACK		
Coffee or tea	10	10 Cal
DINNER		
Beans & Greens Salad (Recipe 20 - page 135)	260	
Whole-grain bread (1 slice)	70	
Baked potato (medium)	100	
Fresh fruit in season (apple, plum, etc)	70	
Water	0	500 Cal
SNACK		
Coffee or tea	10	10 Cal
		1195 Cal

Cooking Daily Menu 21

BREAKFAST	Calories	Totals
Cantaloupe (½ medium)	50	
Fried eggs (2 eggs)	160	
Toasted whole-grain bread (1 slice)	70	
Coffee	10	290 Cal
SNACK		
Yogurt (4 oz, non-fat any flavor)	60	
Coffee or tea	10	70 Cal
LUNCH		
Soup (Appendix B - page 171)	160	
Hard whole-grain roll (medium)	80	
Lettuce & tomato slices	20	
Hot or iced tea	10	270 Cal
SNACK		
Fresh fruit in season (apple, peach, etc)	70	
Coffee or tea	10	80 Cal
DINNER		
Grilled scallops (Recipe 21 - page 136)	210	
Grilled polenta (Recipe 21)	125	
Mushroom-steamed green beans-red onion	45	
Grilled asparagus	10	
Large tossed salad with 1½ Tbsp low-cal dressing	85	
Water	0	475 Cal
SNACK		
Coffee or tea	10	10 Cal
		1195 Cal

Cooking Daily Menu 22

BREAKFAST	Calories	Totals
Orange juice (½ cup)	50	
Oatmeal (½ cup dry) + ½ cup milk + about 15 raisins	220	
Coffee	10	280 Cal
SNACK		
Coffee or tea	10	10 Cal
LUNCH		
Two servings (1 cup) left over Recipe 20 bean salad	260	
Small whole-grain roll	80	
Lettuce & tomato slices	20	
Hot or iced tea	10	370 Cal
SNACK		
Fresh fruit in season (apple, plum, etc)	70	
Coffee or tea	10	80 Cal
DINNER		
Fettuccine (Recipe 22 - page 137)	290	
Large tossed salad with 1½ Tbsp low-cal dressing	85	
Italian or French bread (1 slice)	80	
Water	0	440 Cal
SNACK		
Coffee or tea	10	10 Cal
		1205 Cal

Cooking Daily Menu 23

BREAKFAST	Calories	Totals
Orange juice (½ cup)	50	
Wild blueberry pancakes (Recipe 9 - page 124)	190	
Light syrup (1½ Tbsp)	45	
Coffee	10	295 Cal
SNACK		
Yogurt (4 oz, non-fat any flavor)	60	
Coffee or tea	10	70 Cal
LUNCH		
Salad (3 oz canned tuna, 1 tsp Evoo, onions, celery)	175	
Lettuce & tomato wedges	20	
Rye bread (1 slice)	70	
Fresh fruit in season (apple, pear, etc)	70	
Water with lemon wedge	15	350 Cal
SNACK		
Coffee or tea	10	10 Cal
DINNER		
Barbequed shrimp (Recipe 23 - page 138)	160	
Corn on the cob (medium)	60	
Steamed broccoli (1 cup – after cooking)	50	
Water with lemon wedge	15	315 Cal
SNACK		
Kashi TLC Chewy Granola Bar	140	
Coffee or tea	10	150 Cal
		1190 Cal

Cooking Daily Menu 24

BREAKFAST	Calories	Totals
Fresh orange sliced	75	
Kashi GoLean (1 cup) + ½ cup skim milk + ½ banana	235	
Coffee	10	320 Cal
SNACK		
Fresh fruit in season (apple, plum, etc)	70	
Coffee or tea	10	80 Cal
LUNCH		
Soup (Appendix B - page 171)	140	
Small whole-grain roll	80	
Raw zucchini slices, celery & carrot sticks	20	
Water	0	240 Cal
SNACK		
Coffee or tea	10	10 Cal
DINNER		
Cheeseburger (Recipe 24 - page 139)	370	
Lettuce & sliced tomato	20	
Whole-grain hard roll	140	
Steamed green beans	25	
Pickle spear	0	
Water	0	555 Cal
SNACK		
Coffee or tea	10	10 Cal
		1215 Cal

Cooking Daily Menu 25

BREAKFAST	Calories	Totals
Grapefruit (½)	75	
Scrambled egg	80	
Whole grain toast (1 slice)	70	
Coffee	10	235 Cal
SNACK		
Yogurt (4 oz nonfat, any flavor)	60	
Coffee or tea	10	70 Cal
LUNCH		
Ham (2 oz) with mustard on 2 slices rye bread	300	
Pickle spear	0	
Diet soda or water	0	300 Cal
SNACK		
Fresh fruit in season (apple, plum, etc)	70	
Coffee or tea	10	80 Cal
DINNER		
Baked Sea Bass (Recipe 25 - page 140)	395	
Large tossed salad with 1½ Tbsp low-cal dressing	85	
Water	0	465 Cal
SNACK		
Coffee or tea	10	10 Cal
		1205 Cal

Cooking Daily Menu 26

BREAKFAST	Calories	Totals
Grapefruit (½)	75	
Cheerios (1 cup) + ½ cup skim milk + about 15 raisins	190	
Coffee	10	275 Cal
SNACK		
Coffee or tea	10	10 Cal
LUNCH		
Subway 6" (Turkey Breast, Cheese + veggies)*	230	
Coffee or tea	10	240 Cal
SNACK		
Handful unsalted mixed nuts	100	
Coffee or tea	10	110 Cal
DINNER		
Turkey tenders & veggies (Recipe 26 - page 141)	350	
Spinach (½ cup steamed & drizzled with 1 tsp Evoo)	70	
Romaine lettuce, tomato slices (1 Tbsp low-cal dressing)	45	
Water	0	465 Cal
SNACK		
Nature Valley Crunchy Granola bar	95	
Coffee or tea	10	105 Cal
		1205 Cal

Cooking Daily Menu 27

BREAKFAST	Calories	Totals
Tomato juice (½ cup)	20	
Shredded Wheat (1 cup) + ½ cup skim milk + ½ banana	265	
Coffee	10	295 Cal
SNACK		
Coffee or tea	10	10 Cal
LUNCH		
Roast beef (2 oz) with lettuce sandwich	300	
Hot or iced tea	10	310 Cal
SNACK		
Carrot sticks + ¼ cup low-fat cottage cheese & chives	60	
Coffee or tea	10	70 Cal
DINNER		
Pasta Rapini (Recipe 27 - page 142)	290	
Large tossed green salad with 1½ Tbsp low-cal dressing	85	
Italian or French bread (1 slice)	80	
Hot or iced tea	10	465 Cal
SNACK		
Fresh fruit in season (apple, peach, etc)	70	
Coffee or tea	10	80 Cal
		1200 Cal

Cooking Daily Menu 28

BREAKFAST	Calories	Totals
Cantaloupe (½ medium)	50	
Wheaties (¾ cup) + ½ cup skim milk + ½ banana	190	
Coffee	10	250 Cal
SNACK		
Fresh fruit in season (apple, pear, etc)	70	
Coffee or tea	10	80 Cal
LUNCH		
Soup (Appendix B - page 171)	120	
Turkey (1 oz) on 1 slice of rye bread (½ sandwich)	120	
Water	0	240 Cal
SNACK		
Coffee or tea	10	10 Cal
DINNER		
Grilled Tilapia (Recipe 28 - page 143)	300	
Asparagus spear (6)	25	
Wild rice (½ cup – after cooking)	100	
Large tossed salad with 1½ Tbsp low-cal dressing	85	
Water	0	510 Cal
SNACK		
Popcorn Mini Bag	110	110 Cal
		1200 Cal

Cooking Daily Menu 29

BREAKFAST	Calories	Totals
Orange juice (½ cup)	50	
Soft-boiled egg	80	
Whole-grain toast (1 slice)	70	
Coffee	10	210 Cal
SNACK		
Yogurt (4 oz nonfat, any flavor)	60	
Coffee or tea	10	70 Cal
LUNCH		
Soup (Appendix B - page 171)	220	
Lettuce & tomato wedges + rye bread (1 slice)	60	
Fresh fruit in season – (apple, pear, etc)	70	
Coffee or tea	10	360 Cal
SNACK		
Coffee or tea	10	10 Cal
DINNER		
Low-Cal Beef Stew (Recipe 29 - page 144)	365	
Large tossed salad with 1½ Tbsp low-cal dressing	85	
Small whole-grain roll	80	
Water with lemon wedge	15	545 Cal
SNACK		
Coffee or tea	10	10 Cal
		1205 Cal

Cooking Daily Menu 30

BREAKFAST	Calories	Totals
Fresh sliced orange	75	
Cheerios (1 cup) + ½ cup skim milk + about 15 raisins	190	
Coffee	10	275 Cal
SNACK		
Fresh fruit in season (peach, plum, etc)	70	
Coffee or tea	10	80 Cal
LUNCH		
Cottage cheese (1 cup low fat)	180	
Large tossed salad with 1½ Tbsp low-cal dressing	85	
Small whole-grain roll	80	
Hot or iced tea	10	355 Cal
SNACK		
Handful unsalted mixed nuts	100	100 Cal
DINNER		
Chicken with veggies (Recipe 30 - page 145)	365	
Water with lemon wedge	15	380 Cal
SNACK		
Coffee or tea	10	10 Cal
		1200 Cal

Cooking Daily Menu 31

BREAKFAST	Calories	Totals
Orange juice (½ cup)	50	
Shredded Wheat (1 cup) + ½ cup skim milk + ½ banana	260	
Coffee	10	320 Cal
SNACK		
Coffee or tea	10	10 Cal
LUNCH		
Turkey frank (2 oz) with mustard & relish	150	
Hot dog bun	130	
Diet soda	0	280 Cal
SNACK		
Handful unsalted mixed nuts	100	
Coffee or tea	10	110 Cal
DINNER		
Pasta e Fagioli (Recipe 31 - page 146)	300	
Large tossed salad with 1½ Tbsp low-cal dressing	85	
Italian or French bread (1 slice)	80	
Water with lemon wedge	15	480 Cal
SNACK		
Coffee or tea	10	10 Cal
		1210 Cal

Cooking Daily Menu 32

BREAKFAST	Calories	Totals
Fresh or frozen strawberries (½ cup)	25	
French toasted English Muffin (Recipe 3)	270	
Light syrup (1 Tbsp)	30	
Coffee	10	335 Cal
SNACK		
Yogurt (4 oz nonfat, any flavor)	60	
Coffee or tea	10	70 Cal
LUNCH		
Salad (3 oz canned tuna, 1 tsp Evoo, onions, celery)	175	
Lettuce & tomato wedges	20	
Rye bread (1 slice)	70	
Coffee or tea	10	275 Cal
SNACK		
Coffee or tea	10	10 Cal
DINNER		
Beef Kebob with veggies (Recipe 32- page 147)	390	
Baked potato (medium)	100	
Hot or iced tea	10	500 Cal
SNACK		
Coffee or tea	10	10 Cal
		1200 Cal

Cooking Daily Menu 33

BREAKFAST	Calories	Totals
Orange juice (½ cup)	50	
Kashi GoLean (1 cup) + ½ cup skim milk + ½ banana	235	
Coffee	10	295 Cal
SNACK		
Fresh fruit in season (apple, peach, etc)	70	
Coffee or tea	10	80 Cal
LUNCH		
Subway 6" (Roast Beef, Cheese + veggies)	245	
Diet soda or water	0	245 Cal
SNACK		
Yogurt (4 oz, non-fat, any flavor)	60	60 Cal
DINNER		
Baked Haddock (Recipe 33 - page 148)	420	
Large tossed salad with 1½ Tbsp low-cal dressing	85	
Water with lemon wedge	15	520 Cal
SNACK		
Coffee or tea	10	10 Cal
		1210 Cal

Cooking Daily Menu 34

BREAKFAST	Calories	Totals
Cantaloupe (½ medium)	50	
Perfect egg (Recipe 8a - page 122)	80	
Toasted whole-grain bread (1 slice)	70	
Coffee	10	210 Cal
SNACK		
Yogurt (4 oz nonfat, any flavor)	60	
Coffee or tea	10	70 Cal
LUNCH		
Soup (Appendix B - page 171)	170	
Lettuce & tomato sandwich (1 Tbsp light mayo)	180	
Hot or iced tea	10	360 Cal
SNACK		
Coffee or tea	10	10 Cal
DINNER		
Chicken Cacciatore (Recipe 34a - page 149)	310	
Italian or French bread (1 slice)	80	
Water	0	390 Cal
SNACK		
Blueberry muffin (Recipe 34b - page 150)	145	
Coffee or tea	10	155 Cal
		1195 Cal

Cooking Daily Menu 35

BREAKFAST	Calories	Totals
Grapefruit (½)	75	
Cheerios (1 cup) + ½ cup skim milk + about 15 raisins	190	
Coffee	10	275 Cal
SNACK		
Coffee or tea	10	10 Cal
LUNCH		
Cottage cheese (1 cup low fat)	180	
Large tossed salad with 1½ Tbsp low-cal dressing	85	
Diet soda or water	0	265 Cal
SNACK		
Coffee or tea	10	10 Cal
DINNER		
Poached Cod (Recipe 35 - page 151)	275	
Grilled potatoes	100	
Grilled cherry tomatoes	45	
Spinach (½ cup) steamed with garlic, drizzled with Evoo	50	
Water with lemon wedge	15	485 Cal
SNACK		
Blueberry muffin	145	
Coffee or tea	10	155 Cal
		1200 Cal

Cooking Daily Menu 36

BREAKFAST	Calories	Totals
Fresh orange sliced	75	
Soft-boiled egg	80	
Whole-grain toast (1 slice)	70	
Coffee	10	235 Cal
SNACK		
Yogurt (4 oz nonfat, any flavor)	60	
Coffee or tea	10	70 Cal
LUNCH		
Salad – 3 oz canned salmon, 1 tsp Evoo, onions & celery	200	
Lettuce & tomato wedges	20	
Rye bread (1 slice)	70	
Water	0	290 Cal
SNACK		
Fresh fruit in season (apple, plum, etc)	70	
Coffee or tea	10	80 Cal
DINNER		
Chicken Piccata (Recipe 36 - page 152)	270	
Brown rice (½ cup – after cooking)	100	
Large tossed salad with 1½ Tbsp low-cal dressing	85	
Small bunch of grapes	65	
Water	0	520 Cal
SNACK		
Coffee or tea	10	10 Cal
		1205 Cal

Cooking Daily Menu 37

BREAKFAST	Calories	Totals
Cantaloupe (½ medium)	50	
Wheaties (¾ cup) + ½ cup skim milk + ½ sliced banana	190	
Coffee	10	250 Cal
SNACK		
Coffee or tea	10	10 Cal
LUNCH		
Ham (2 oz) with mustard on 2 slices rye bread	290	
Pickle spear	0	
Hot or iced tea	10	300 Cal
SNACK		
Handful unsalted mixed nuts	100	
Coffee or tea	10	110 Cal
DINNER		
Beans and Greens Salad (Recipe 37 - page 153)	260	
Whole-grain bread (1 slice)	70	
Baked potato (medium)	100	
Water with lemon wedge	15	515 Cal
SNACK		
Coffee or tea	10	10 Cal
		1195 Cal

Cooking Daily Menu 38

BREAKFAST	Calories	Totals
Fresh or frozen strawberries (1 cup)	25	
French toasted English Muffin (Recipe 3 - page 117)	270	
Light syrup (1 Tbsp)	30	
Coffee	10	335 Cal
SNACK		
Yogurt (4 oz nonfat, any flavor)	60	
Coffee or tea	10	70 Cal
LUNCH		
Soup (Appendix B - page 171)	110	
BLT sandwich (2 slices turkey bacon, Tbsp light mayo)	245	
Pickle spear	0	
Hot or iced tea	10	355 Cal
SNACK		
Coffee or tea	10	10 Cal
DINNER		
Pan-fried Sole (Recipe 38 - page 154)	325	
Large tossed salad with 1½ Tbsp low-cal dressing	85	
Water with lemon wedge	15	420 Cal
SNACK		
Coffee or tea	10	10 Cal
		1205 Cal

Cooking Daily Menu 39

BREAKFAST	Calories	Totals
Grapefruit (½)	75	
Cheerios (1 cup) + ½ cup skim milk + about 15 raisins	190	
Coffee	10	275 Cal
## SNACK		
Fresh fruit in season (peach, plum, etc)	70	
Coffee or tea	10	80 Cal
## LUNCH		
Cottage cheese (1 cup low fat)	180	
Large tossed salad with 1½ Tbsp low-cal dressing	85	
Hot or iced tea	10	275 Cal
## SNACK		
Handful unsalted mixed nuts	100	
Coffee or tea	10	110 Cal
## DINNER		
Beef steak strips (Recipe 39 - page 155)	330	
Steamed spinach (½ cup)	25	
Baked potato (medium)	100	
Water	0	455 Cal
## SNACK		
Coffee or tea	10	10 Cal
		1205 Cal

Cooking Daily Menu 40

BREAKFAST	Calories	Totals
Cantaloupe (½ medium)	50	
Fried egg	80	
Toasted whole-grain bread (1 slice)	70	
Coffee	10	210 Cal
SNACK		
Yogurt (4 oz nonfat, any flavor)	60	60 Cal
LUNCH		
Soup (Appendix B - page 171)	200	
Hard whole-grain roll (medium)	80	
Lettuce & tomato slices	20	
Small bunch of grapes	65	
Water	0	365 Cal
SNACK		
Coffee or tea	10	10 Cal
DINNER		
Grilled scallops (Recipe 40 - page 156)	210	
Grilled polenta (Recipe 40)	125	
Mushroom-steamed green beans (Recipe 40)	45	
Grilled asparagus (Recipe 40)	10	
Large tossed salad with 1½ Tbsp low-cal dressing	85	
Water	0	475 Cal
SNACK		
Fresh fruit in season (apple, peach, etc)	70	
Coffee or tea	10	80 Cal
		1200 Cal

BREAKFAST	Calories	Totals
Tomato juice (½ cup)	**20**	
Kashi GoLean (1 cup) + ½ cup skim milk + ½ banana	**235**	
Coffee	**10**	**265 Cal**
SNACK		
Coffee or tea	**10**	**10 Cal**
LUNCH		
Subway 6" (Turkey Breast, Cheese + veggies)	**230**	
Diet soda (or water)	**0**	**230 Cal**
SNACK		
Coffee or tea	**10**	**10 Cal**
DINNER		
Grilled pork chop with orange (Recipe 41 - page 157)	**470**	
Wild rice (¼ cup – after cooking)	**50**	
Asparagus (7 spear cooked & drained)	**20**	
Water	**0**	**540 Cal**
SNACK		
Blueberry muffin	**145**	
Coffee or tea	**10**	**155 Cal**
		1210 Cal

Cooking Daily Menu 42

BREAKFAST	Calories	Totals
Cantaloupe (½ medium)	50	
Smoothie (Recipe 42a - page 158)	220	
Coffee	10	280 Cal
SNACK		
Coffee or tea	10	10 Cal
LUNCH		
Turkey breast (2 oz) on 2 slices bread	245	
Lettuce, tomato and 1 Tbsp light mayo	35	
Pickle spear	0	
Diet soda or water	0	280 Cal
SNACK		
Coffee or tea	10	10 Cal
DINNER		
Pasta Salad (Recipe 42b - page 159)	370	
Italian or French bread (1 slice)	80	
Water with lemon wedge	15	465 Cal
SNACK		
Blueberry muffin	145	
Coffee or tea	10	155 Cal
		1200 Cal

Cooking Daily Menu 43

BREAKFAST	Calories	Totals
Fresh or frozen strawberries (½ cup)	25	
French toasted English Muffin (Recipe 3 - page 117)	270	
Light syrup (1 Tbsp)	30	
Coffee	10	335 Cal
SNACK		
Yogurt (4 oz nonfat, any flavor)	60	
Coffee or tea	10	70 Cal
LUNCH		
Salad (3 oz canned tuna, 1 tsp Evoo, onions, celery)	175	
Lettuce & tomato wedges	20	
Rye bread (1 slice)	70	
Water	0	265 Cal
SNACK		
Fresh fruit in season (apple, pear, etc)	70	70 Cal
DINNER		
Beef Burgundy (Recipe 43 - page 160)	350	
Large tossed salad with 1½ Tbsp low-cal dressing	85	
Water with lemon wedge	15	450 Cal
SNACK		
Coffee or tea	10	10 Cal
		1200 Cal

Cooking Daily Menu 44

BREAKFAST	Calories	Totals
Grapefruit (½)	75	
Scrambled egg	80	
Whole-grain toast (1 slice)	70	
Coffee	10	235 Cal
SNACK		
Yogurt (4 oz nonfat, any flavor)	60	
Coffee or tea	10	70 Cal
LUNCH		
Ham (2 oz) with mustard on 2 slices bread	290	
Pickle spear	0	
Water	0	290 Cal
SNACK		
Coffee or tea	10	10 Cal
DINNER		
Chicken cutlet (Recipe 44 - page 161)	450	
One small baked potato	50	
Large tossed salad with 1½ Tbsp low-cal dressing*	85	
Water	0	585 Cal
* Note: Much of salad is on the plate with cutlet.		
SNACK		
Coffee or tea	10	10 Cal
		1200 Cal

Cooking Daily Menu 45

BREAKFAST	Calories	Totals
Grapefruit (½)	75	
Cheerios (1 cup) + ½ cup skim milk	160	
Coffee	10	245 Cal
SNACK		
Coffee or tea	10	10 Cal
LUNCH		
Cottage cheese (1 cup low fat)	180	
Tossed salad with 1½ Tbsp low-cal dressing	70	
Water	0	250 Cal
SNACK		
Coffee or tea	10	10 Cal
DINNER		
Personal-Size Meat Loaf (Recipe 45 - page 162**)**	410	
Brown rice (½ cup – after cooking)	100	
Green beans - steamed	30	
Water	0	540 Cal
SNACK		
Blueberry muffin	145	
Coffee or tea	10	155 Cal
		1210 Cal

Cooking Daily Menu 46

BREAKFAST	Calories	Totals
Cantaloupe (½ medium)	50	
Fried egg	80	
Whole-grain toast (2 slices)	140	
Coffee	10	280 Cal
SNACK		
Yogurt (6 oz, nonfat, any flavor)	90	
Coffee or tea	10	100 Cal
LUNCH		
Soup (Appendix B - page 171)	160	
Whole-grain bread (1 slice)	70	
Hot or iced tea	10	240 Cal
SNACK		
Fresh fruit in season (apple, plum, etc)	70	
Coffee or tea	10	80 Cal
DINNER		
Crab Cakes (Recipe 46 - page 163)	320	
Baked potato (medium)	100	
Large tossed salad with 1½ Tbsp low-cal dressing	70	
Water	0	490 Cal
SNACK		
Coffee or tea	10	10 Cal
		1200 Cal

Cooking Daily Menu 47

BREAKFAST	Calories	Totals
Grapefruit (½)	75	
Cheerios (1 cup) + ½ cup skim milk	160	
Coffee	10	245 Cal
SNACK		
Fresh fruit in season (apple, plum, etc)	70	
Coffee or tea	10	80 Cal
LUNCH		
Salad (3 oz canned tuna, 1 tsp Evoo, onions, celery)	175	
Lettuce & tomato wedges	20	
Rye bread (1 slice)	70	
Coffee or tea	10	275 Cal
SNACK		
Handful unsalted mixed nuts	100	
Coffee or tea	10	110 Cal
DINNER		
Black-Eyed Peas (Recipe 47 - page 164)	280	
Brown rice (½ cup – after cooking)	100	
Small whole-grain roll	80	
Water with lemon wedge	10	470 Cal
SNACK		
Coffee or tea	10	10 Cal
		1190 Cal

Cooking Daily Menu 48

BREAKFAST	Calories	Totals
Orange juice (½ cup)	50	
Shredded Wheat (1 cup) + ½ cup skim milk + ½ banana	260	
Coffee	10	320 Cal
SNACK		
Coffee or tea	10	10 Cal
LUNCH		
Turkey frank (2 oz) with mustard & relish	150	
Hot-dog bun	130	
Diet soda or water	0	280 Cal
SNACK		
Coffee or tea	10	10 Cal
DINNER		
Pasta Pomodoro (Recipe 48 - page 165)	420	
Large tossed salad with 1½ Tbsp low-cal dressing	70	
Italian or French bread (1 slice)	80	
Water with lemon wedge	10	580 Cal
SNACK		
Coffee or tea	10	10 Cal
		1210 Cal

Cooking Daily Menu 49

BREAKFAST	Calories	Totals
Cantaloupe (½ medium)	50	
Wheaties (¾ cup) + ½ cup skim milk + ½ banana	190	
Coffee	10	250 Cal
SNACK		
Fresh fruit in season (apple, plum, etc)	70	
Coffee or tea	10	80 Cal
LUNCH		
Turkey frank (2 oz) with mustard & relish	150	
Hot-dog bun	130	
Hot or iced tea	10	290 Cal
SNACK		
Celery sticks + ¼ cup low-fat cottage cheese & chives	60	
Coffee or tea	10	70 Cal
DINNER		
Healthy Frittata (Recipe 49 - page 166)	320	
Large tossed salad with 1½ Tbsp low-cal dressing	70	
Small whole-grain roll	80	
Water with lemon wedge	10	500 Cal
SNACK		
Coffee or tea	10	10 Cal
		1190 Cal

Cooking Daily Menu 50

BREAKFAST	Calories	Totals
Orange juice (½ cup)	50	
Shredded Wheat (1 cup) + ½ cup skim milk + ½ banana	265	
Coffee	10	325 Cal
SNACK		
Coffee or tea	10	10 Cal
LUNCH		
Subway 6" (Ham, Cheese + veggies)	260	
Fresh fruit in season (apple, plum, etc)	70	
Hot or iced tea	10	340 Cal
SNACK		
Fresh fruit in season (apple, plum, etc)	70	
Coffee or tea	10	80 Cal
DINNER		
Mediterranean Chicken (Recipe 50 - page 167)	200	
Spaghetti squash (1 cup steamed & drizzled with 1 tsp	90	
Green beans (¼ lb – steamed)	25	
Small whole-grain roll	80	
Hot or iced tea	10	405 Cal
SNACK		
Coffee or tea	10	10 Cal
		1200 Cal

Recipe 1

Chicken with Peppers & Onions

    4 boneless and skinless chicken breasts (5 oz each)

Coat the chicken breasts in a bottled barbeque sauce. Prepare medium-hot fire on well-oiled grill. Place breasts on grill, turning them every 4 minutes, for 10 to 12 minutes, or until done. (To check if breasts are done, the meat should be moist and white with no sign of pink when you cut into the breast.) Salt and pepper to taste.

    2 medium red peppers, sliced

    1 medium onion, sliced

Place peppers and onions in pan with 2 tablespoons fat-free chicken stock. Sauté until stock is reduced. Spray pan lightly with non-stick cooking oil and cook another 2 minutes. Salt and pepper to taste.

Serves 4. About 250 Calories per serving (for chicken only).

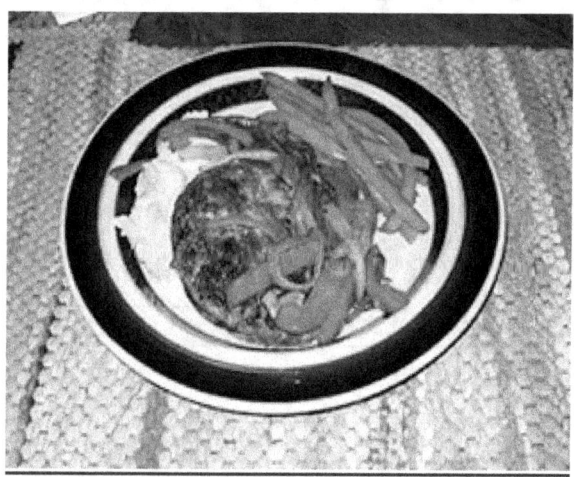

Diet Tip of the Day: Weight Loss – take it one step, one meal, one workout, one day at a time. Just think of where you'll be in 60 days!

Recipe 2

Baked Herb-Crusted Cod

4   cod fish fillets (4 to 5 ounces each)
2   tablespoons flour
2   tablespoons cornmeal
2   tablespoons minced fresh herbs
2   teaspoons lemon juice

Sprinkle cod with lemon juice. Mix flour, cornmeal and herbs and dust the cod with the cornmeal-herb mixture. Bake in oven at 375 °F for 10 minutes. Add salt and black pepper to taste.

Serves 4. One serving is about 230 Calories (for cod only).

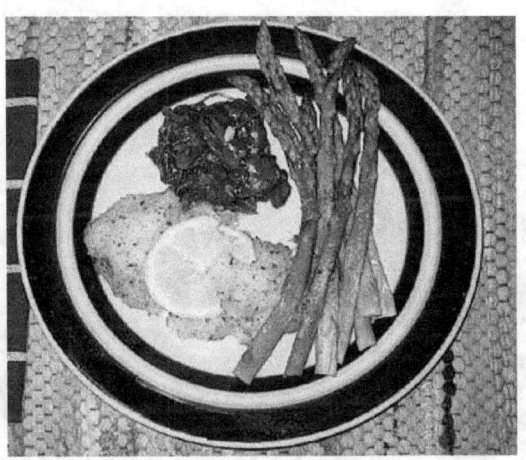

Diet Tip of the Day:. A **reducing diet is best supervised by a physician**. This is especially true when a great deal of weight needs to be lost, or if you have an ailment or a history of medical problems.

Recipe 3

French-Toasted English Muffin

    6 whole grain light English muffins, sliced in half
    4 eggs
    2 cups skim milk
    2 teaspoons vanilla
    A dash of cinnamon

In a medium bowl, beat together eggs and skim milk. Add vanilla and cinnamon. Slice English muffins into halves and saturate slices in egg mixture. In a non-stick skillet coated with cooking spray, cook muffins until both sides are golden brown. Dust lightly with confectionary sugar. Serve hot or keep in an oven or warmer at 200 °F until ready to plate.

Serves 4. Three English muffin slices per serving. Serving is 270 Calories.

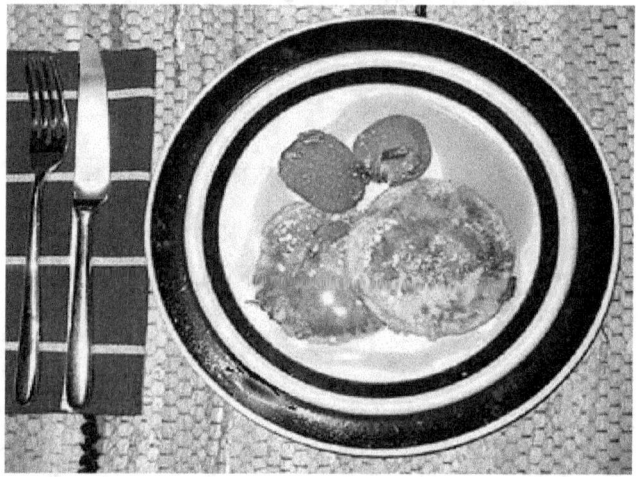

Diet Tip of the Day: "Eat Slowly" This is especially vital when you are trying to lose weight. If you are someone who eats fast, who finishes before everyone else at the table, you are not giving yourself a chance to feel full. While everyone else is still eating, you either sit there and pick, or you have seconds, taking in extra calories you could avoid if you would just slow down.

Recipe 4

Carrie's Low-Cal Meat Loaf

  ½ pound ground white meat turkey
  ½ pound ground beef (about 60% lean)
  1 large egg
  ½ cup skim milk
  ¼ cup bread crumbs
  ¼ cup ketchup
  ¼ cup chopped carrots
  ¼ cup chopped onion

In a medium bowl, combine all ingredients. Add salt and pepper to taste.
Mix until blended and form into a loaf. Place loaf into oven preheated to 350
°F. Bake until an instant-read thermometer inserted in the center of the loaf
reads 160 °F. This should take about one hour.

Shown below is meat loaf, acorn squash (baked with 1 teaspoon of maple
syrup). Also shown is steamed spinach drizzled with extra-virgin olive oil.
Serves 5. About 290 Calories per serving (for meat loaf only). Note: reserve
half a serving of the meat loaf which is to be eaten for lunch on Day 6.

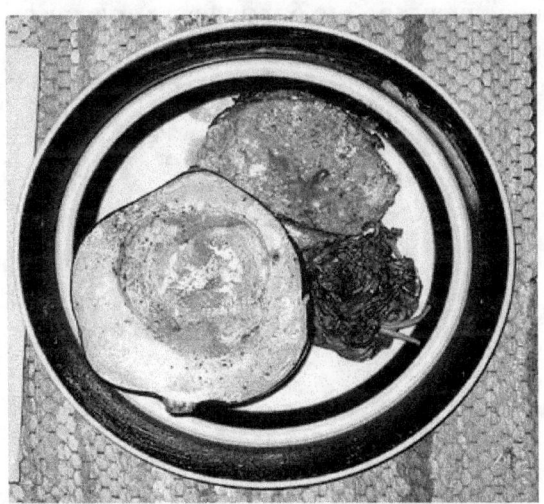

Diet Tip of the Day: **Take a daily multi-vitamin/mineral supplement.**
This is very important when you're on a diet – as a kind of insurance policy.

Recipe 5

Veal with Mushrooms & Tomato

½ pound spaghetti
¾ pound veal cutlets
8 ounces sliced mushrooms
2 tablespoon olive oil, divided
2 tablespoons flour
3 green onions, small, sliced
½ cup chicken broth
14.5-ounce can diced tomatoes

Pound veal to about ¼-inch thickness. Rinse, pat dry and cut into 2-inch pieces. Heat 1 tablespoon olive oil in large nonstick skillet over medium heat. Add mushrooms and cook, stirring, until lightly browned. Remove and set aside.

Season veal with salt and pepper and coat lightly with flour. Add remaining olive oil to skillet and cook veal over medium heat for about 2 minutes on each side, or until browned. Add the green onions and cook for 1 minute longer. Add chicken broth and cook, uncovered, for 5 minutes. Add tomatoes; cover and simmer for 3 to 5 minutes. Serve over spaghetti cooked per package directions.

Serves 4   520 Calories per serving (includes spaghetti)

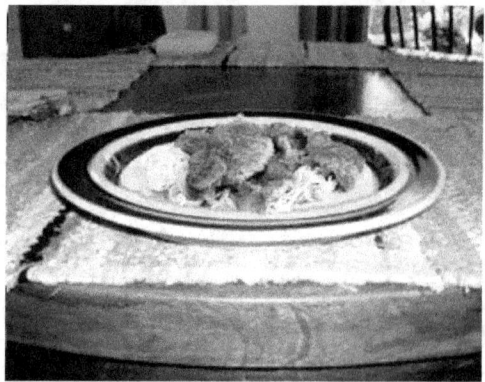

Diet Tip of the Day: Successful weight loss and subsequent weight maintenance **requires knowledge, desire and discipline**. Avoid the latest fad diets. Instead, take the time to develop a true understanding of weight control and then change your eating and activity habits accordingly.

Recipe 6

Grandma's Pizza

The following is a pizza recipe used by Gail Johnson's Italian grandmother. She was from a small mountain village located between Rome and Naples.

Pizza dough: To save time use prepared dough, preferably whole grain. To start, flour a large cutting board. Divide one pound of prepared pizza dough into four parts. Roll out each dough ball as thin as possible.

Tomato sauce: Sauté ½ small onion, chopped fine, in 1 teaspoon olive oil. Add two finely chopped garlic cloves, 1½ cups chopped plum tomatoes and ½ teaspoon chopped fresh oregano. Stir and cook about 5 minutes on a low flame.

Pizza preparation & cooking: On each pizza, spread evenly ¼ cup of the tomato sauce. Add ½ ounce of shredded part-skim mozzarella cheese, 1 teaspoon Parmesan cheese, 3 slices of a Portobello mushroom, some torn fresh basil, and drizzle with extra-virgin olive oil. Put pizzas on a pan and place in 475 °F oven for about 15 to 20 minutes, or until crust is crisp and cheese is just melting. (Freeze left over sauce for use on Day 13.)

<u>**Serves 4**</u>.   Each pizza contains approximately 350 Calories.

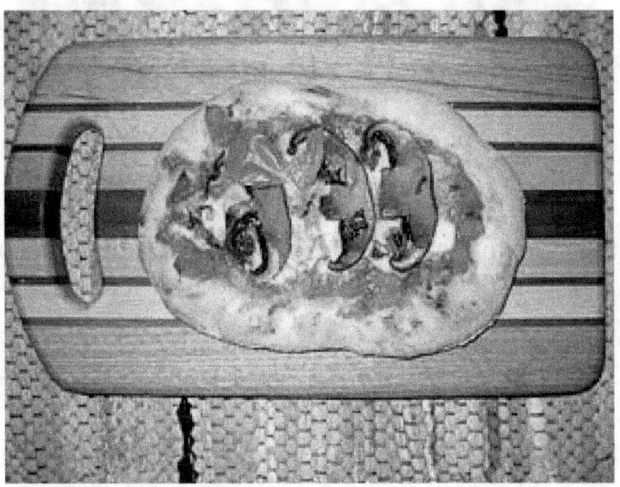

<u>**Diet Tip of the Day:**</u> For **life-long weight control** take a vigorous 30 to 60 minute walk everyday! That's right – everyday. Make exercise a nonflexible top priority part of your life. When it comes to exercise the key words are consistent, persistent, unyielding, dogged. Get the point?

Recipe 7

Baked Salmon with Salsa

This is a simple, straight-forward recipe. The advantage of a simple recipe is there are no hidden calories.

    4 5 oz salmon fillets
    6 tablespoons bottled tomato-pepper salsa

Brown salmon fillets in non-stick pan and then place them in a baking dish. Cook fillets in an oven preheated to 350 ℉ for about 10 minutes. Plate the salmon. Stir bottled tomato-pepper salsa and spoon it over the salmon. **Serves 4**. One salmon fillet is about 215 Calories.

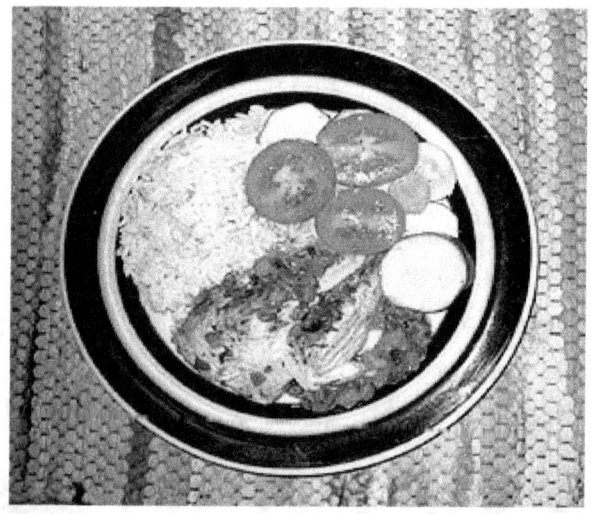

Diet Tip of the Day: Hunger is your body's way of telling you that you need calories. But **when you're done eating, you should feel better – satisfied but not stuffed**.

Recipe 8a

<u>The Perfect Egg</u>

Why perfect? Because it's cooked with no added fat, and a perfect egg is low calorie, nutritious and delicious. It takes about one minute to prepare - and there is virtually no clean up afterwards. It's perfect for busy people on the go, or for anyone who wants a quick, easy nutritious breakfast. For best results cook the egg in a well-glazed (shinny and smooth), microwave safe, 4-inch diameter cup with straight sides and a flat bottom.

<u>Step 1</u>: In the microwave-safe cup, beat an extra-large egg with about 2 teaspoons of added water for easy clean up.

<u>Step 2</u>: Place cup in microwave at full power for approximately 40 seconds, or until the egg begins to rise, gets fluffy and most of the added water has evaporated. (The actually cooking time will depend on how powerful your microwave is.) Salt and pepper to taste.

<u>Step 3</u>: Remove cup from the microwave and slide the egg onto a slice of whole-grain toast, (or as shown in the photo on a toasted bagel). Salt and pepper to taste.

<u>**Serves 1**</u>: Perfect Egg is 80 Calories. When a Perfect Egg is eaten with a slice of whole grain toast the calorie total is about 150.

Step 1

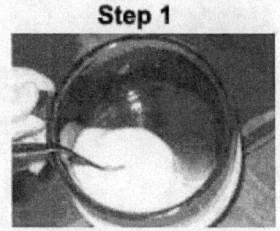

Egg Well Beaten

Step 3

Step 2

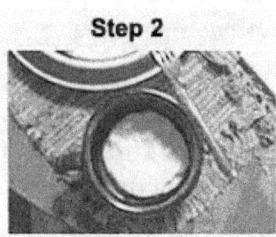

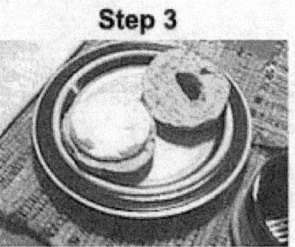

Hot From Microwave   **Perfect Egg on Bagel**

Recipe 8b

Veggie Burger

Vegetable-based burgers can be purchased at your local supermarket. Patties of a veggie burger are made from either vegetables, soy, nuts, mushrooms, textured vegetable protein, dairy, or a combination of these foods.

In the U.S., two popular veggie burgers are the Boca Burger and Gardenburger. The Boca Burger is made chiefly from soy protein and grain gluten. (Boca Burger patties are 2.5 oz each and range from 60 to 60 Calories.) The original Gardenburger is made from mushrooms, onions, brown rice, rolled oats, cheese, and spices. (Gardenburger patties are 2.5 oz each and about 100 Calories.)

To prepare, follow package directions. The version shown below has an added slice of low-fat cheddar cheese. The lettuce, tomato and ketchup shown actually add very few extra calories.

The veggie burger patty plus low-fat cheese amounts to approximately 150 Calories. Add a seeded roll and the total rises to 290 Calories.

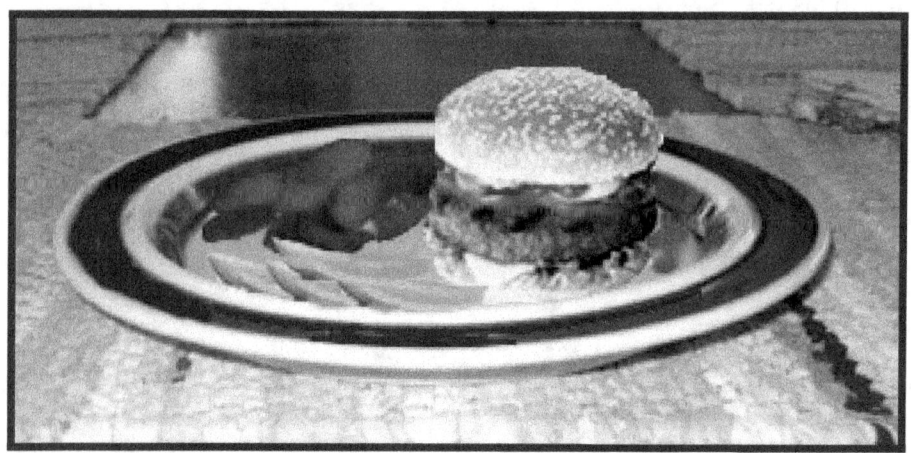

Diet Tip of the Day: **Drink lots of water** – about 8 glasses per day when you're trying to lose weight. Add a slice of lemon to make it more interesting. Often, when you think you're hungry, you are just thirsty. So, next time you crave a snack, drink some water first and see if that does it for you.

Recipe 9

<u>Wild Blueberry Pancakes</u>

This recipe makes a relatively low calorie, wholesome batch of delicious wild blueberry-whole grain-buttermilk pancakes.

1 cup whole-grain flour
1   cup buttermilk
1 egg
1 tablespoon vegetable oil
1 teaspoon baking powder
½ teaspoon baking soda

Stir ingredients until blended. Add ¾ cup fresh of frozen blueberries and gently stir. Using medium heat, preheat a non-stick skillet coated with cooking spray. Pour slightly less than ¼ cup of batter onto skillet per pancake. Cook slowly until bubbles break on surface of pancake. Turn and cook until other side is lightly browned.

Makes 8 pancakes. Pictured below are wild-blueberry pancakes with two slices of turkey bacon.
Serves 4. Each pancake is about 95 Calories

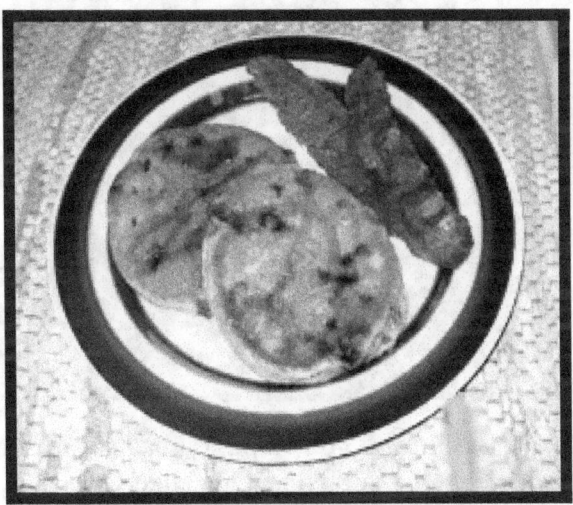

Bacon allowable only on 1,500 and 1,800 Calorie diets.

<u>Diet Tip of the Day:</u> Most experts associate eating a substantial breakfast with successful weight loss.

Recipe 10

Artichoke-Bean Salad

    19-ounce can white kidney beans
    10 artichoke hearts, quartered
    ⅓ cup chopped oregano
    ⅓ cup chopped parsley
    3 cloves garlic, chopped
    1 lemon, juiced

Combine ingredients in medium-size bowl. Stir in ¼ cup extra-virgin olive oil. Salt and black pepper to taste.

Serves 6. Approximately 190 Calories per serving.

Pictured on the plate below is the <u>artichoke-bean salad</u> as a side dish with two grilled chicken sausage links, tomato salsa and steamed green beans. Incidentally, this artichoke-bean combination over mixed salad greens served with a whole-grain bread makes a delicious, nutritious and reasonable low-calorie main course.

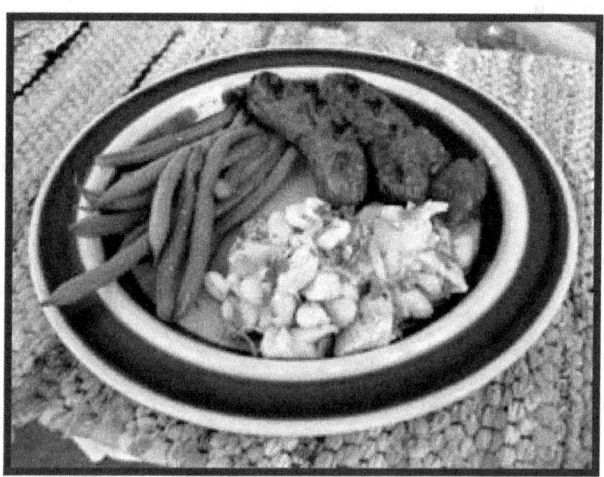

<u>Diet Tip of the Day:</u> Before you go to a **party**, have a small meal, such as a hardboiled egg, an apple, and a thirst quencher (like water, tea, seltzer, or diet soda). This will take the edge off your appetite and make it easier to resist the high-calorie goodies.

Pasta with Marinara Sauce

Prepare the sauce as you did for the Recipe 6 - Pizza (page 119). But because the pizza sauce is a bit too thick, we add ¼ cup of pasta liquid to thin it. (The spiral pasta profile shown below is called fusilli, a very popular pasta shape because all those ridges hold buckets of tomato sauce.)

   ½ pound <u>whole-grain</u> pasta
   ¼ teaspoon salt

Prepare the marinara tomato sauce as per Day 6 sauce but dilute it with ¼ cup of today's pasta liquid.

Bring 2 quarts of lightly salted water to a boil. Add pasta and stir occasionally (to keep pasta from sticking to the bottom of the pot). Keep water boiling and cook until pasta are "al dente." (Cooking time is approximately 9 minutes.) Drain pasta, add marinara sauce and serve hot.
<u>Serves 4.</u> One serving is about 225 Calories.

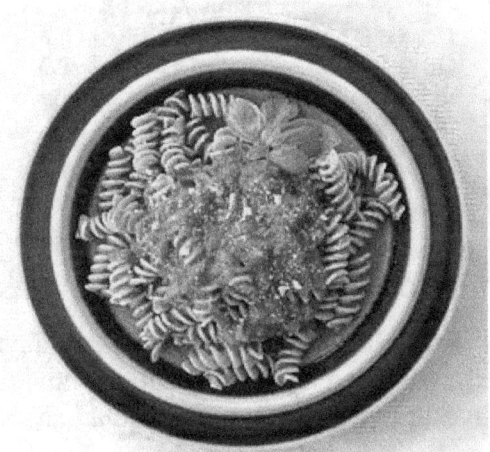

<u>Diet Tip of the Day:</u> **Beware of alcoholic beverages**. Beer has about 13 Calories per ounce, wine 25 Calories per ounce and whiskey a whopping 71 Calories per ounce.

Recipe 12

<u>London Broil</u>

   1 lb boneless flank steak about ¾" thick, fat trimmed
   1 clove garlic
   1 teaspoon dry oregano

Rub each side of the flank steak with garlic. Season with oregano, salt and pepper to taste. Prepare a large non-stick skillet over high heat. Steak should sizzle when placed on hot skillet. Sear steak on one side for about 5 minutes; then turn and sear other side for about 4 minutes, or until done to preference. Check the center by making small incision. Carve into ¼-inch slices.
<u>Serves 4</u>. About 320 Calories per serving (for meat only).

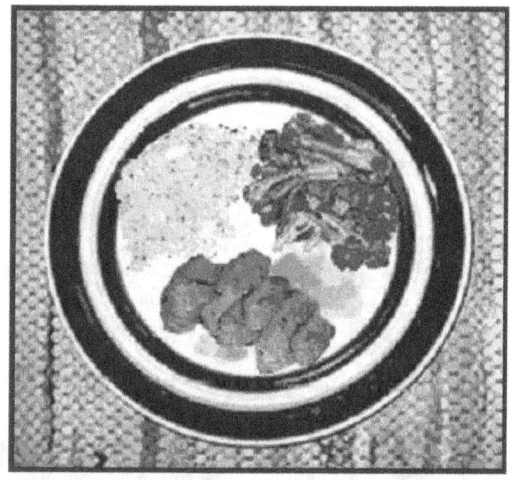

<u>Diet Tip of the Day:</u> Stay Busy. Most people will do anything to avoid work, housework, yard work, exercise, etc. But any kind of work burns a lot more calories than just sitting! Whatever it is you are avoiding – just go do it!

Recipe 13

__Red Snapper with Special Sauce__

  4   4-ounce red snapper fillets (salmon fillets okay)
  ½ cup white wine
  ½ cup non-fat yogurt mixed with ¼ cup mustard
  ½ pound green beans
  ¾ pint cherry tomatoes (about 20), halved
  4 teaspoons olive oil
  ¾ cup wild rice, brown rice and grain berry mix.

Brown fillets in non-stick pan. Place fillets skin side down in baking dish
coated with non-stick spray. Add white wine and cook in oven preheated to
350 ºF for about 15 minutes . Spoon pan juices over fillets. Salt and pepper to
taste.

Place green beans in skillet. Add ¼-inch of water and cook over medium heat
until water boils off. Add cherry tomatoes and olive oil. Stir well and sauté
for a few minutes. (If desired, season with fresh rosemary and oregano.) Salt
and pepper to taste.

Prepare rice mix per package directions

Plate red snapper fillet and spoon over yogurt-mustard sauce. Add green
beans and tomato mix and the wild rice mix. Serve hot.

__Serves 4.__ One plate consisting of one snapper fillet (215 Calories) with green
beans and tomato mix (75 Calories) and wild rice (160 Calories) totals 450
Calories.

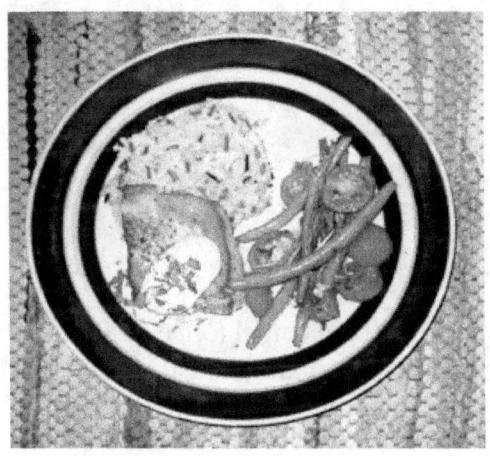

Recipe 14

Cajun Chicken Salad

This is a perfect after-work, quick, nutritious and delicious dinner.

    4 boneless and skinless chicken breasts - about 5 oz each
    4 teaspoons of bottled Cajun herb-spice mix
    8 ounces mixed salad greens
    ¾ pint cherry tomatoes (about 20), halved
    12 pitted black olives
    2 tablespoons bottled light salad dressing

Brush chicken breasts lightly with olive oil. Roll breasts in Cajun herb-spice mix.

Brown breasts on non-stick oven-proof skillet. After breasts are brown, put skillet in 350 °F oven for approximately 15 minutes, or until done. (When the breasts are done, the meat should be moist and white with no sign of pink.) Cut breasts into ½-inch slices.

Serve hot or keep in an oven or warmer at 200 °F until ready to plate. Place chicken slices over a bed of mixed salad greens. Add tomatoes, olives and two tablespoons of your favorite low-calorie salad dressing.
Serves 4. 330 Calories per serving

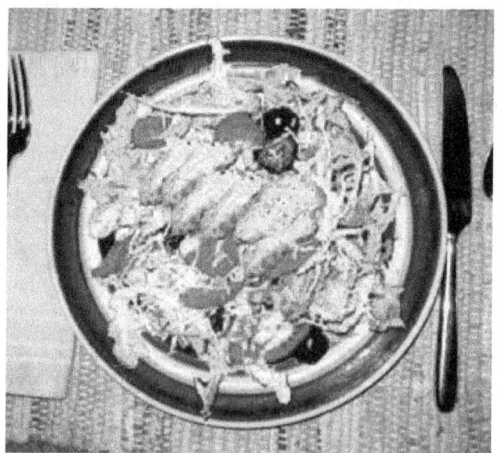

Diet Tip of the Day: Hot or cold cereal topped with fruit, and fat-free milk makes a nutritious, relatively low-calorie meal anytime.

Recipe 15

Grilled Swordfish

1¼ pounds swordfish
1 bottle citrus-herb marinade
¾ pint cherry tomatoes (about 20), halved
4 medium potatoes
2 cups fresh spinach
1 teaspoon rosemary & juice of ¼ lemon
2 teaspoon extra-virgin olive oil, divided

Steam spinach with garlic and drizzle with about 1 teaspoon extra-virgin olive oil.

Cut potatoes in medium-size pieces and sprinkle with lemon juice, add rosemary, salt and black pepper. Place potatoes on grill for about 10 minutes, turning occasionally.

Toss cherry tomatoes in remaining extra-virgin olive oil. Add fresh oregano, salt and black pepper. Place on heavy-duty aluminum foil, seal and grill for about 3 minutes.

Marinade swordfish in citrus-herb vinaigrette. Grill on hot fire for about 5 minutes on one side and 3 minutes on the other, or until done as desired.
Serves 4. One plate of grilled swordfish (250 Calories) with potatoes (100 Calories), cherry tomatoes (45 Calories) and steamed spinach (50 Calories) totals 445 Calories.

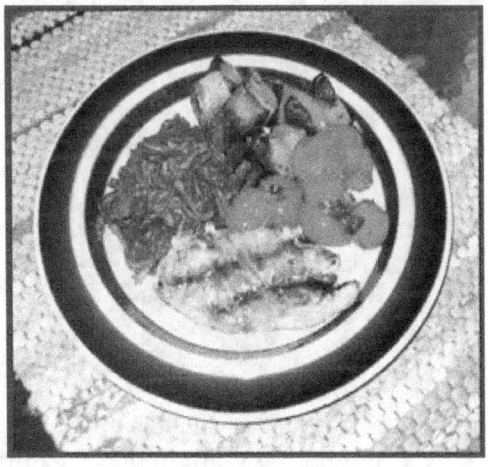

Recipe 16

Quick Pasta alla Puttanesca

This famous pasta dish originated in Naples Italy. Puttanesca means "ladies of the night." Although the exact origin of the name is unclear, one thing is clear: It's delicious! Here is one of many recipe versions.

½ pound spaghetti (whole grain preferred)
20 black or green pitted olives
14.5-oz can diced tomatoes
4 oz tomato sauce
2 tablespoon extra-virgin olive oil
3 cloves of garlic, chopped
1 tablespoon dried minced onion
½ teaspoon crushed red pepper flakes
1 tablespoon capers drained and rinsed
¼ cup currants

Cook spaghetti according to package directions. Drain and return spaghetti to pot; add a teaspoon extra-virgin olive oil and toss to coat.

Heat remaining olive oil in large skillet over medium-high heat. Add red pepper flakes; cook and stir 1 to 2 minutes or until sizzling. Add onion and garlic; cook and stir 1 minute. Add canned tomatoes with juice, tomato sauce, olives, currants and capers. Cook over medium-high heat, stirring frequently, until sauce is heated through.

Serves 4. About 345 Calories per serving

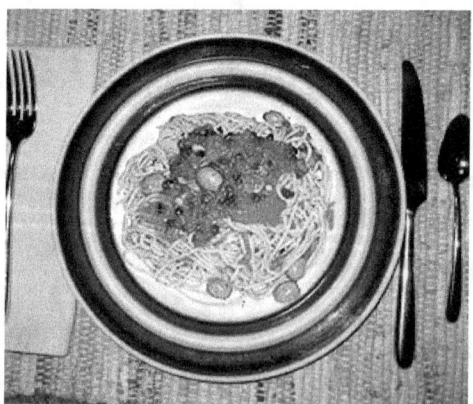

Diet Tip of the Day: Dilute fruit juices, such as apple juice, orange, etc. with water. This cuts the flavor slightly but really reduces calorie content.

Recipe 17

<u>Shrimp & Spinach Salad</u>

   2 pounds shrimp in shell
   ½ pound small green beans, trimmed
   ½ pound baby spinach leaves
   2 tablespoon lemon juice
   ¼ cup extra-virgin olive oil
   2 teaspoon minced fresh dill
   1 tablespoon minced green onion

To make vinaigrette, combine lemon juice, olive oil, dill, salt and black pepper to taste and whisk until blended. Stir in minced onion and set aside. Steam green beans and set aside.

Peel, de-vein and butterfly shrimp. Place shrimp in a bowl and add water to cover. Add 1 teaspoon of salt, and let stand for 10 minutes. Drain, rinse, drain again, and dry. Arrange shrimp in broiling pan without a rack. Brush shrimp with a little of the vinaigrette and place under preheated broiler, about 3 inches from heat. Broil about 3 to 4 minutes, turning shrimp once, or until both sides turn pink.

Remove shrimp from broiler and add remaining vinaigrette and green beans to the broiling pan. Stir to coat shrimp and beans with vinaigrette. Pour warm vinaigrette over spinach and toss quickly. Plate the spinach and arrange shrimp and green beans on top.
<u>Serves 4</u>. 310 Calories per serving.

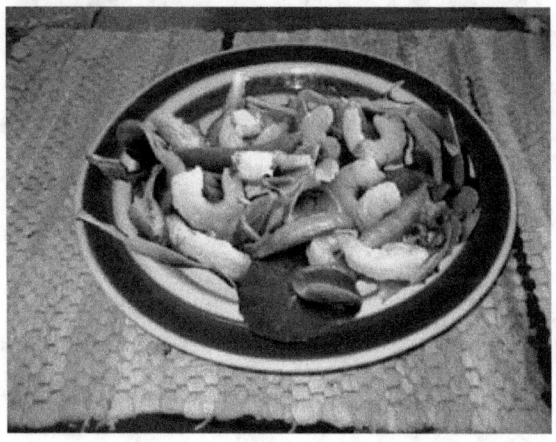

Recipe 18

Pan-Broiled Hanger Steak

    1¼ pounds hanger steak, well trimmed of fat
    ¼ cup lime juice
    8 small new potatoes, peeled and halved
    ½ pint cherry tomatoes (about 15), halved

Season both sides of steak with salt and pepper and place in sealable plastic bag with lime juice. Refrigerate for about one hour.

Boil potatoes about 10 minutes. Rinse in cold water. Sauté potatoes in small amount of vegetable oil over medium-high heat until brown.

Sauté cherry tomatoes in small amount of olive oil over medium-high heat until skin begins to crack. Season with chopped fresh basil.

Heat a skillet over medium-high heat. Sear hanger steak on one side for about 5 minutes. Turn over and sear other side approximately 5 minutes (for medium done). Pour off any fat that may have accumulated. Cut into ½-inch slices.

Serves 4. About 320 Calories per serving (for the hanger steak only)

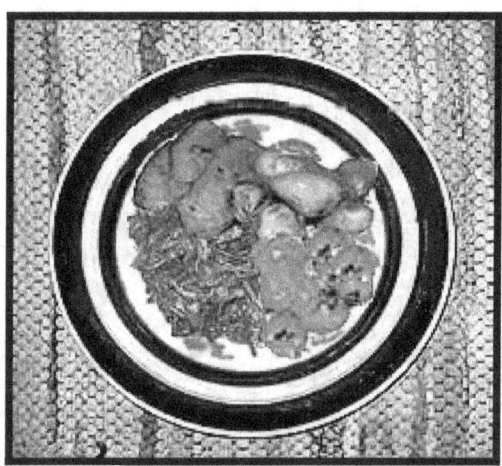

Diet Tip of the Day: If you go to a **party**, don't stand near the food! Be aware of the temptation. Make the effort, and you'll find you eat less.

Recipe 19 (This is a side dish)

Four-Bean Plus Salad

Note that the total caloric value of the salad will change very little, if the proportions of the bean varieties and corn are varied – according to taste.
½ cup canned red kidney beans, drained and rinsed
½ cup canned black beans, drained and rinsed
½ cup canned chick peas, drained and rinsed
½ cup canned cannelloni beans, drained and rinsed
½ cup canned corn, drained
1 small red pepper, chopped
1 small green pepper, chopped
2 tablespoons extra-virgin olive oil
2 tablespoons lemon juice
In a large bowl mix red kidney beans, black beans, chick peas, cannelloni beans, corn and chopped red and green peppers. Stir in olive oil and lemon juice and plate.
Serves about 6. One serving is ½ cup – with about 135 Calories per serving

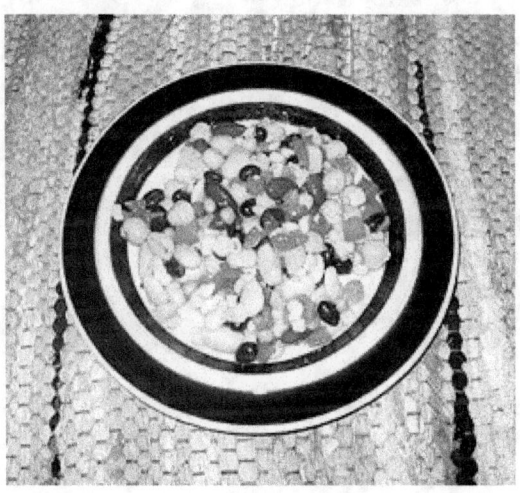

Diet Tip of the Day: Vigorous exercise doesn't necessarily stimulate you to overeat. Just the opposite. In many cases, exercise actually helps curb your appetite – immediately following a workout.

Recipe 20

<u>Beans & Greens Salad</u>

⅓ cup chopped oregano
⅓ cup chopped parsley
3 cloves garlic, chopped
1 lemon, juiced

Prepare dressing by combining above ingredients and stirring in ¼ cup extra-virgin olive oil. Salt and black pepper to taste.

½ pound mesclun mix
¼ pound green beans
19-oz can garbanzo beans (chickpeas)

Arrange mesclun mix, garbanzo beans and green beans on large platter.
Drizzle dressing over beans and greens.
<u>Serves 4</u>. Approximately 260 Calories per serving.

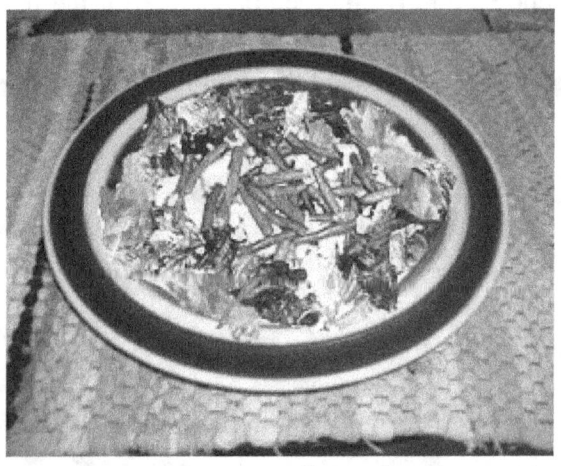

<u>Diet Tip of the Day:</u> Beans are a wonderful food but **beans are an incomplete protein**. If however beans are eaten with a whole-grain bread, the combination forms a complete protein – just as complete and nutritious as meat, poultry, or fish.

Grilled Scallops &Polenta

- 1 pound sea scallops
- ¾ cup polenta cornmeal
- ¾ cup skim milk
- 1 medium portobello mushroom
- ½ pound green beans
- ¼ cup chopped red onion
- 16 asparagus spear
- 1 teaspoon extra-virgin olive oil

Bring 1½ cups of water and skim milk to rapid boil. Add salt to taste and slowly add polenta while stirring. Reduce heat. Continue stirring until desired consistency is reached. Pour polenta into lightly greased pan. After polenta has cooled cover and refrigerate. Cut chilled polenta into 4 pieces. Grill on medium-hot fire – about two minutes on each side.

Brush portobello mushroom and asparagus spear with olive oil and place on grill for about 3 minutes on each side.

Grill scallops on medium-hot fire. Turn after two minutes or when first side turns opaque. Grill until second side turns opaque – about another 2 minutes. Don't overcook but test a scallop by cutting to make sure it's cooked through. Salt and pepper to taste.

<u>Serves 4.</u> The food on the plate pictured below totals about 380 Calories.

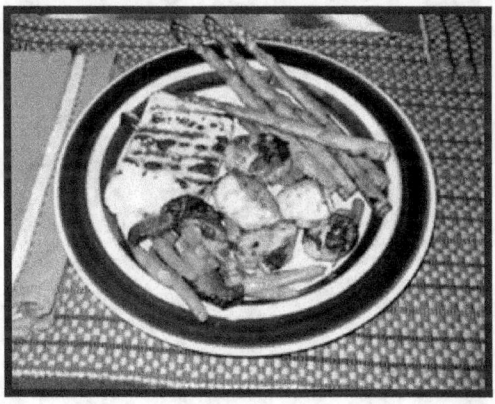

<u>Diet Tip of the Day:</u> To have better control of what you eat **bring your lunch to work**.

Recipe 22

Fettuccine in Summer Sauce

This sauce is often served in the summer because it's lighter than what is usually dished up with pasta. But despite its name the sauce is wonderful year round.

½ lb fettuccine
8 oz fresh asparagus, trimmed & cut in 2-inch pieces
¾ pint cherry tomatoes (about 20), halved
2 Tbsp plus 1 tsp extra-virgin olive oil, divided
2 cloves of garlic, chopped
½ small onion, diced
Cook fettuccine according to package directions. Drain and return pasta to pot; add a teaspoon of the olive oil and toss to coat. Meanwhile steam asparagus and drain.

In large skillet over medium-high heat, sauté cherry tomatoes in remaining 2 tablespoons of olive oil until skin begins to crack. Add onion and cook until translucent. Stir in garlic. Thin sauce with pasta liquid to desired consistency. Toss cooked pasta and asparagus into sauce and serve immediately.
Serves 4. About 290 Calories per serving

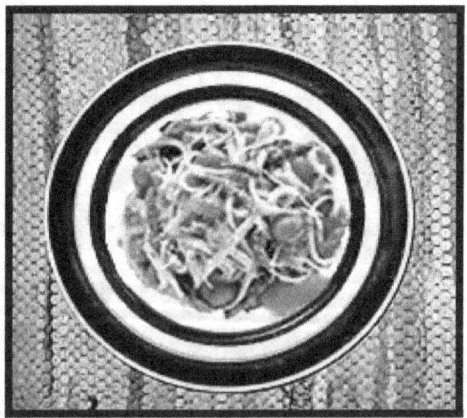

Diet Tip of the Day: A major weight-loss fallacy is that you can **get rid of abdominal fat** by working your abdominal muscles. This is based on the incorrect belief that fat is eliminated from a particular part of your body if you engage the muscles underneath that layer of fat. No such luck.

Recipe 23

<u>Barbequed Shrimp & Corn</u>

1½ pounds large shrimp, peeled and de-veined
3 Tbsp of your favorite bottled barbeque sauce
4 medium ears of corn
Pour barbeque sauce into shallow bowl. Toss shrimp in barbeque sauce to coat. Place shrimp on medium-hot grill. Turn shrimp after about two minutes or when shrimp turn pink. Grill until second side turns pink – approximately another 2 minutes. Don't overcook but test a shrimp by cutting to make sure it is cooked through. Salt and pepper to taste. Serve hot or at room temperature.
<u>Serves 4</u>. About 160 Calories per serving (shrimp only).

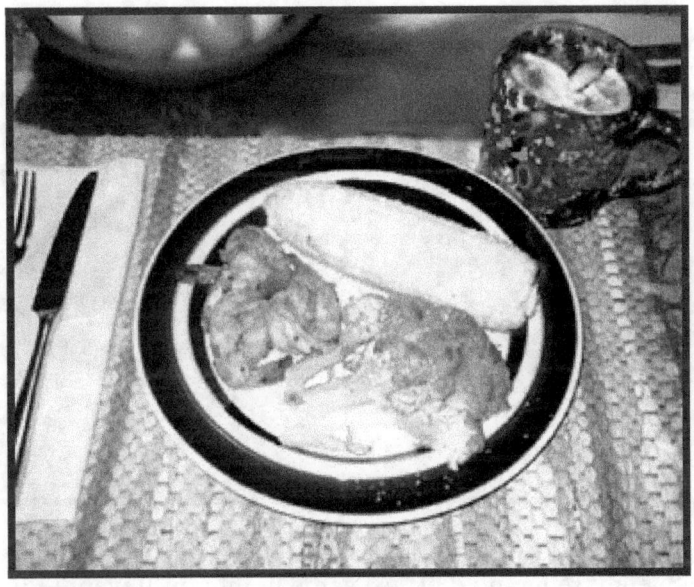

<u>Diet Tip of the Day:</u> A very **important weight-profile parameter** is your waist-to-hip ratio. Health risks for heart attack and stroke increase considerably for men with a ratio above 1.0 and for women with a ratio above 0.8. To calculate your ratio, measure your waist size (at its narrowest circumference) and divide it by your hip size (at the widest section).

Recipe 24

Cheeseburger Heaven

There's really not much to grilling hamburgers. The ideal meat for a juicy burger is ground chuck with about 20% fat, but we are talking diet here. So we opt for leaner, much leaner meat.

    1¼ pounds ground sirloin (95% lean)
    4 thin slices low-fat American cheese

Mix ground beef in large bowl. Salt and pepper to taste. Divide into 4 equal portions and form burgers about 1-inch thick.

Cook burgers over a hot fire on charcoal or gas-fired grill. For medium, cook about 4 minutes on each side. Top with slice of cheese. Add lettuce and tomato. Season to taste.

Serves 4. About 370 Calories per serving (cheeseburger only).

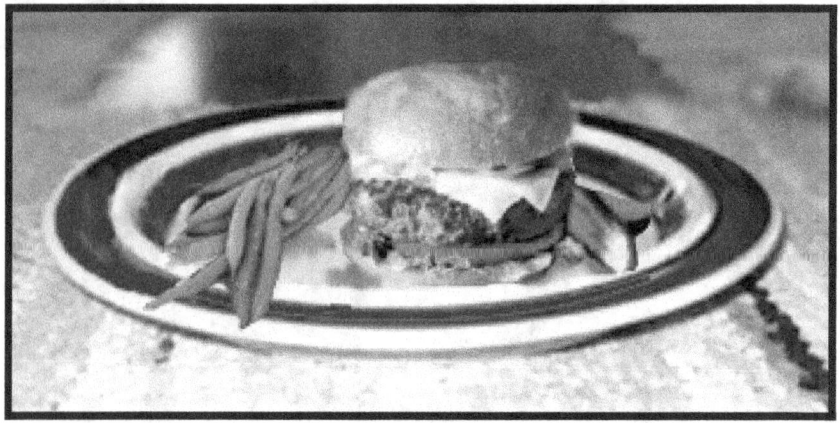

Diet Tip of the Day: **Plan to be on a diet the rest of your life**. Not necessarily a weight reducing diet. At some point you'll want to just maintain your weight. But you will still need to continue to make good healthy food choices – and not slip back to your old eating habits.

Recipe 25

Tina's Baked Sea Bass

    4 4-ounce Chilean sea bass fillets
    ½ pound green beans
    ¾ pint cherry tomatoes (about 20)
    ¾ cup brown rice (prepare per package directions)

Sea Bass: Dust filets with flour. Dip in egg wash & then Panko bread crumbs. Place fillets in baking dish coated with non-stick spray. Bake about 15 minutes in oven preheated to 350 °F.

Green Beans & Tomato: Place green beans in skillet. Add ¼-inch of water and cook over medium heat until water boils off. Add cherry tomatoes and olive oil. Stir well and sauté for a few minutes. Season with fresh rosemary and oregano.

Brown Rice-Pesto mix: Prepare brown rice per package directions. Add 4 teaspoons packaged "green" pesto. Mix thoroughly.

Red Pepper Sauce: Blend one roasted red pepper (skinned), ½ cup non-fat yogurt, 1 tsp lemon juice, 1 Tbsp olive oil, 1 Tbsp chili sauce, and a dash of Worcestershire sauce.

Serves 4. One plate consisting of one sea bass fillet with spooned over red pepper sauce (150 Calories), green beans & tomato mix (75 Calories), brown rice-pesto mix (120 Calories) and half ear of corn (50 Calories) – totals about 395 Calories.

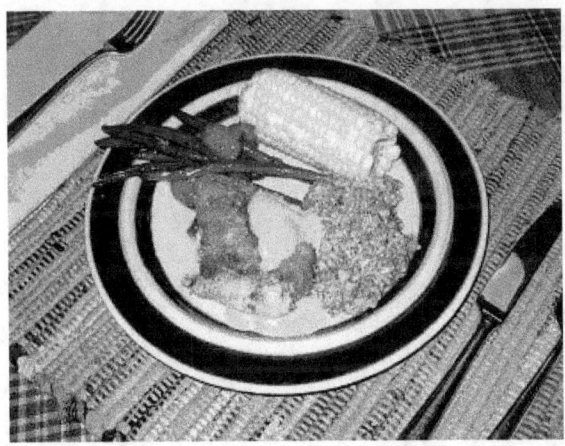

<u>Diet Tip of the Day:</u> Protein foods make you **feel full longer** and help prevent overeating.

Recipe 26

Turkey Tenders & Vegetables

 2 turkey breast tenderloins (about 1½ lb)
 1 medium eggplant (about ¾ lb)
 ¾ pound yellow (summer) squash
 2 medium plum tomatoes, quartered

Marinade: Whisk in a bowl 2 tsp lemon zest, ¼ cup lemon juice, 2 Tbsp olive oil, 1 Tbsp chopped garlic, 1 Tbsp chopped rosemary, ¼ tsp salt and a pinch of black pepper. Put marinade and turkey breasts in large re-sealable plastic bag. Refrigerate about 45 minutes

Slice eggplant and squash lengthwise about ½-inch thick. Place with tomatoes on a baking sheet coated with a nonstick spray.

Grill turkey breasts approximately 7 to 9 minutes per side, or until an instant-read thermometer inserted from the side to middle registers 160°F. Slice turkey and set aside.

Grill eggplant and zucchini about 4 minutes per side, or until just tender. Grill tomatoes about 2 minutes per side, or until charred but not soft. Cut vegetables bite-size and toss with remaining marinade. Serve with sliced turkey.

Serves 4. About 350 Calories per serving (includes turkey and veggies)

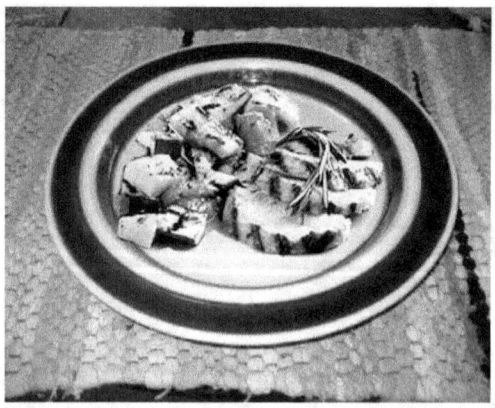

Diet Tip of the Day: It's a lot easier to eat 1000 Calories than it is to burn 1000 Calories exercising. So a stroll after dinner isn't going to offset the calories you ingested eating a Big Mac plus fries.

Recipe 27

<u>Pasta Rapini</u>

    2 cloves garlic - coarsely chopped
    1½ cups of crushed San Marzano tomatoes
    2 cups Rapini (broccoli rabe)
    1 tablespoon crushed red pepper flakes (optional)
    ½ pound medium-sized whole grain pasta

<u>Tomato Sauce:</u> In large pan, sauté two tablespoons olive oil over medium-high heat. Add the garlic and sauté until translucent (but not browned). Add crushed San Marzano tomatoes (use plum tomatoes if San Marzano are not available) and bring to a boil. Reduce heat to low and simmer for about 30 minutes or until cooked. Season with salt and pepper. Set aside.

<u>Rapini:</u> Discard the tough stems and slice into 2-inch pieces. Bring a pot of water to a boil. Add Rapini (a variety of the vegetable broccoli rabe) and 1 tablespoon salt. Blanch Rapini about 5 minutes or until slightly cooked but still crunchy at stems. Drain, set aside and cover.

Cook pasta according to package instructions until al dente. Three minutes before pasta is ready, add the Rapini to the sauté pan (containing the tomato sauce). Heat mixture over medium heat. Drain pasta and add it to the pan with the Rapini and tomatoes. Add hot pepper flakes (optional) and toss for 1 to 2 minutes over high heat. Drizzle lightly with extra virgin olive oil and plate. Delicious!

<u>Serves 4</u>. About 290 Calories per serving

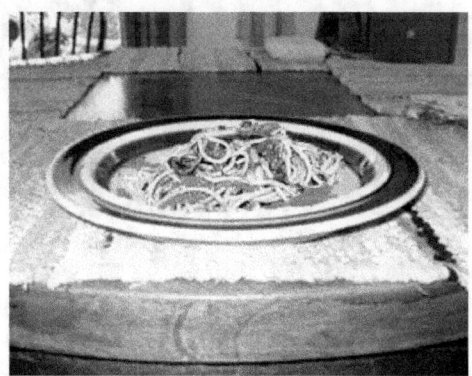

<u>**Diet Tip of the Day:**</u> Keep a daily food log to **record everything you eat**. For some people it really works wonders.

Recipe 28

Grilled Tilapia

Tilapia is a mild, white fish that inhabits fresh water. This fish has very low levels of mercury because it's fast-growing, short-lived, and mostly eats a vegetarian diet. According to the Monterey Bay Aquarium, choose tilapia farmed in the U.S., in environmentally friendly systems. "Avoid" farmed tilapia from China and Taiwan, where pollution and weak management are a problem.

4 Tilapia filets (about 6 ounces each)

Marinade: ¾ cup olive oil, ½ lemon, juiced, 1 tablespoons oregano, ½ teaspoon black pepper, ¼ cup red wine vinegar, ½ cup finely chopped parsley, 2 cloves garlic, minced and 2 dashes Tabasco (optional).

Combine all ingredients (except filets) in a large re-sealable plastic bag and shake well. Then place fish filets in the marinade for 30 minutes. Remove fillets from marinade and cook on hot grill for approximately 2 to 3 minutes per side.

Serves 4. About 300 Calories per serving (fish only)

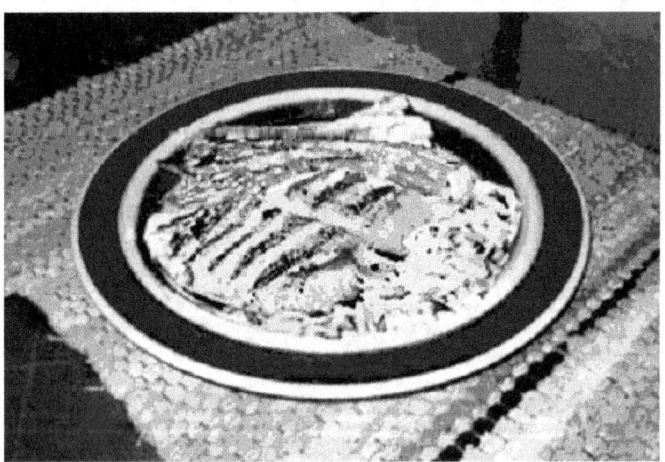

Photo shows two fish filets. Actual serving size is one filet.

Diet Tip of the Day: One serving of asparagus can provide you with 66% of your daily folate needs. Folate is a B-vitamin which is involved with cellular division, and therefore aids the development of a baby's nervous system.

Recipe 29

Lo-Cal Beef Stew

½ lb beef stew meat, fat trimmed & cut in 1" cubes
2 celery stalks diced
1 medium onion diced
3 large carrots cut into large chunks
3 large boiling potatoes, peeled & cut in chunks
½ up green beans
1 container beef stock (low sodium)
2 tablespoons of flour, and 1 tablespoon of olive oil
½ teaspoon dried herbs, and 1 bay leaf

Season meat with ½ teaspoon dried herbs, salt and pepper. In a Dutch oven, add olive oil and heat until warm. Add meat, diced onion and celery and cook over medium heat about 5 minutes. Add enough beef stock to cover meat. Bring to a boil. Reduce heat, add bay leaf, cover and simmer over low heat until meat is fork tender (about 1½ hours). Add potatoes and carrots. Cover and cook until vegetables are tender (about 30 min). Add green beans and cook an additional 10 min. Skim off any fat from the surface.

In a small bowl, add small amount of water to 2 tablespoons of flour – and stir. Pour the flour-water mixture into the stew and stir until a thick gravy forms. Taste and adjust seasoning. Spoon approximately ¼ of the stew in each plate.

Serves 4. About 365 Calories per serving

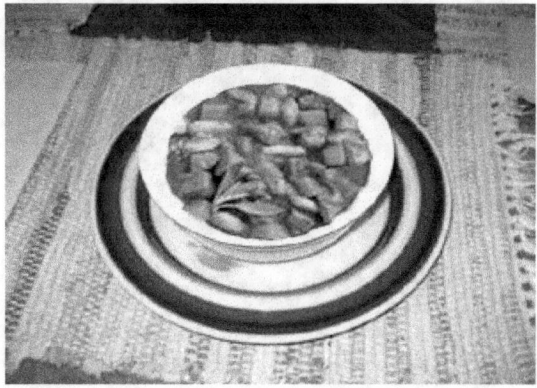

Diet Tip of the Day: **Free-range** animals get more exercise and eat a natural diet, so their meat is usually lower in fat and calories than farm-raised cattle.

Recipe 30

Chicken with Veggies

  4 boneless, skinless chicken breast halves (about 5 oz each)
12 broccoli florets
  1 bunch of asparagus
  2 ripe medium-size tomatoes
  2 tablespoons Lo-Cal (light) salad dressing

Place evenly cut broccoli and asparagus spear in a microwave-safe pan, add a little water to bottom of the pan and top with microwave-safe plastic wrap. (Be sure to pull back one corner of the plastic topper so some steam can escape.) Check veggies periodically and take them out of the microwave when they reach desired softness.

Season chicken breasts evenly with salt and pepper. Heat a large nonstick skillet over medium-high heat. Coat pan with cooking spray. Cook chicken about 4 minutes on each side or until no pink remains.

For each serving, plate one chicken breast and a portion of the steamed broccoli and asparagus. Add one-half of a tomato cut into pieces. Drizzle about 2 tablespoons of a light salad dressing that contains no more than 50 Calories in 2 tablespoons.

Serves 4: One serving of chicken breast halve, veggies & dressing is about 365 Calories.

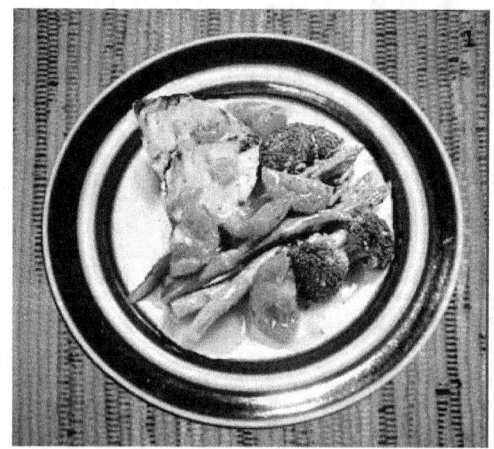

Shown drizzled with Light Thousand Island dressing.

Diet Tip of the Day: Steaming in a microwave oven is one of the best ways to cook veggies so they retain nutrients. Another advantage is the cooking adds no fat or sodium.

Pasta e Fagioli

This is one variation of a traditional, nutritious peasant dish served all over Italy.

14.5-oz can whole tomatoes with juice, crushed
14.5-oz can cannellini beans, drained
1 cup of any tube-shaped pasta
2 tablespoon olive oil
1 medium onion, diced
2 cloves garlic, minced
1 stalk celery, finely chopped
3 cups chicken stock
2 cups fresh baby spinach or escarole
1 tsp dried basil
½ teaspoon dried oregano
2 Tbsp fresh parsley, chopped

Heat olive oil, onion and celery in large saucepan over medium heat. Sauté until onions are golden brown. Add garlic and stir constantly for one minute. Pour in tomatoes and their juices and bring to a boil. Add beans and chicken stock and return to a boil. Stir in spinach (or escarole) and seasonings. Simmer for about 5 minutes. Add pasta and cook about 15 minutes or until pasta is tender but firm. If needed, thin soup with hot water.

Ladle into soup bowls. Garnish with grated Parmesan cheese. Salt and pepper to taste.
Serves 4. About 300 Calories per serving.

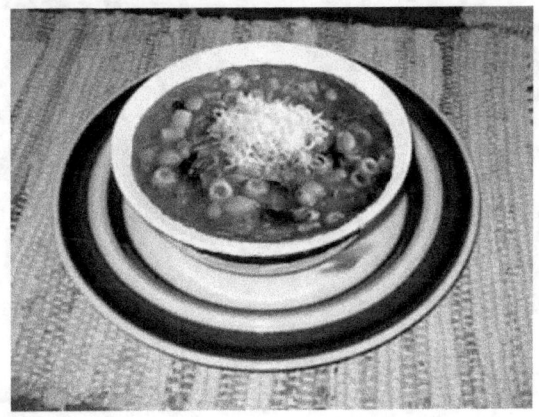

Recipe 32

Beef Kebob

  1 lb boneless beef tenderloin steaks, 1" thick
  8 ounces medium mushrooms
  2 medium bell peppers (any color), cut in pieces
Marinate ingredients:
  2 tablespoons olive oil
  1 tablespoon chopped fresh oregano
  2 cloves garlic, minced
  ½ teaspoon ground black pepper

Cut beef steak into 1-inch square pieces. Combine marinate ingredients in large bowl. Add beef, mushrooms and bell pepper pieces. Toss to coat. Cover bowl and refrigerate for about two hours. Thread beef and vegetable pieces onto eight 12-inch metal skewers.

Grill kebobs over medium-high heat for 8 to 10 minutes, turning occasionally. Check center of meat with a small incision to determine when the meat is done.

Microwave a one-pound package of frozen mixed vegetables. Plate two kebob skewers and about one-quarter of the mixed veggies.
Serves 4. One plate consisting of two kebob skewers (350 Calories) plus ¼ pound of mixed green vegetables (40 Calories) totals about 390 Calories.

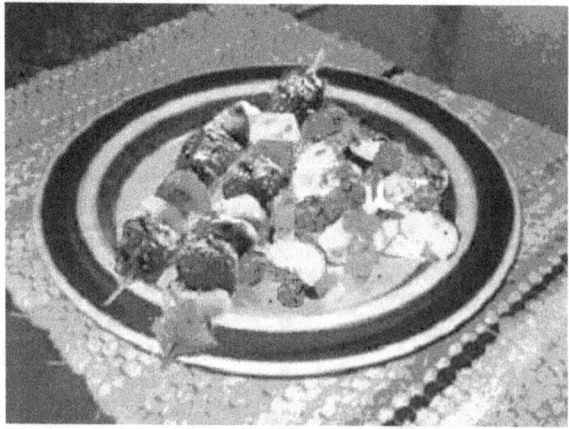

Diet Tip of the Day: Remember your stomach is about the size of your fist. So it doesn't take much food to fill it comfortably.

Recipe 33

<u>Baked Haddock</u>

  4　4-oz haddock fillets (or salmon fillets)
  ½　cup white wine
  ½　cup non-fat yogurt mixed with ¼ cup pureed roasted red pepper
  ½　pound green beans
  ¾　pint cherry tomatoes (about 20)
  1　tablespoon olive oil
  ¾　cup bulgur, prepared per package directions

Lightly dust fillets with flour. Dip in beaten egg white and then in Panko bread crumbs. Brown fillets in non-stick pan. Place fillets skin side down in baking dish coated with non-stick spray. Add white wine and cook in oven preheated to 350 °F for about 15 minutes. Spoon pan juices over fillets. Salt and pepper to taste.

Place green beans in skillet. Add ¼-inch of water and cook over medium heat until water boils off. Add cherry tomatoes and olive oil. Stir well and sauté for a few minutes. Season with fresh rosemary and oregano. Salt and pepper to taste.

Plate haddock fillet and spoon over yogurt-red pepper sauce. Garnish with fresh parsley. Add green beans & tomato mix and the bulgur. Serve hot.

Serves 4. One plate consisting of a haddock fillet (215 Calories) with green beans & tomato mix (65 Calories) and bulgur (140 Calories) totals 420 Calories.

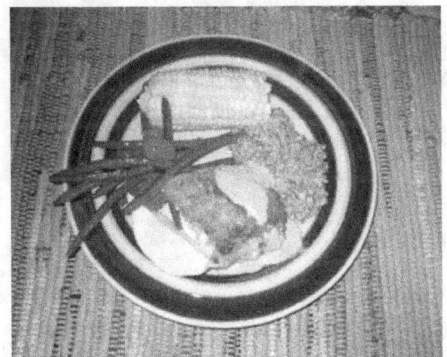

Note that corn-on-the-cob is only for the 1,800 Calorie diet.

Diet Tip of the Day: It's much easier to stay with an exercise program when it's done in tandem. So enlist a friend to be your exercise buddy.

Chicken Cacciatore

- ¾ lb skinless, boneless chicken breast halves
- ¼ lb of your favorite pasta
- ½ cup chopped onion
- ½ cup chopped green bell pepper
- 14.5-ounce can chopped tomatoes, drained
- 8-ounce can tomato sauce
- 1½ teaspoons Italian seasoning
- ⅓ cup sliced ripe olives
- ⅛ teaspoon black pepper

Cut chicken breasts into small pieces. Spray a large heavy skillet with olive oil flavored cooking spray.

Sauté chicken, onion and green pepper for 6 to 8 minutes. Stir in drained tomatoes and tomato sauce. Add Italian seasoning, olives and ⅛ teaspoon ground black pepper. Mix well to combine. Lower heat and simmer for 15 to 20 minutes, stirring occasionally.

Cook pasta per package directions. Ladle chicken and sauce over pasta and serve immediately.
Serves 4. About 310 Calories per serving

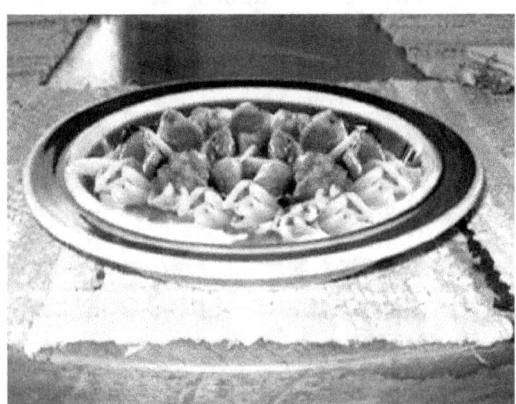

Diet Tip of the Day: Inevitably, you're going to be faced with a stressful situation. Instead of turning to food for comfort, be prepared with some non-food tactics that work for you, such as listening to music, reading, writing in a journal, or meditating.

Recipe 34b

Dawn's Blueberry Muffins

Wholesome whole-grain blueberry muffins just like grandma used to make.
Serve them at breakfast, or as a nutritious dessert, or a wonderful snack.
(Make a dozen. Have one today and store the remainder in your freezer until
they are called for again later in the diet.)

4 ounces bran flakes
¼ cup sugar
1¼ cups whole grain flour
1 teaspoon baking soda
¼ teaspoon baking powder
¼ teaspoon salt
½ cup blueberries (fresh or frozen)
1 egg, beaten
1 cup buttermilk
¼ cup vegetable oil

Preheat oven to 400 °F. Coat muffin tins with nonstick cooking spray. In a
bowl combine dry ingredients. In another bowl combine wet ingredients and
mix thoroughly. Add wet ingredients to dry ingredients and mix until just
blended. Do not over mix. Gently fold in blueberries. Spoon batter into
muffin tins until two-thirds full. Bake 15 minutes or until muffin tops are
golden brown.
Yield is 12 Muffins, 145 Calories each

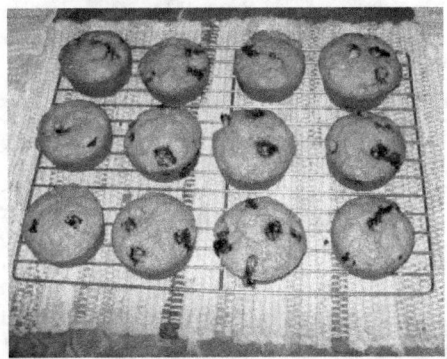

Diet Tip of the Day: **Acquire a good low-calorie cookbook**. Be sure the
recipes cover breakfast, lunch and dinner, and all the recipes contain
nutritional information, especially the calories per serving.

Recipe 35

Poached Cod in Tomato Broth

2   cups dry white wine
1   cup clam juice
2   cans (14.5-ounce) diced tomatoes, drained
1   small onion, diced
1   garlic clove, minced
½   tsp dried parsley, or sprigs of fresh parsley
1   bay leaf
12 black olives, pitted and halved
4   cod fish fillets (about 6 ounces each)

Note that sole, flounder, halibut or haddock may be substituted for cod.

Use a pan large enough to hold the fish in a single layer. Place all the ingredients except the fish in the pan. Over high heat, bring poaching liquid to a boil (pan uncovered). Reduce heat and simmer the liquid another 6 minutes.

Carefully place the fish filets in the liquid. Cover the pan and reduce heat until liquid is just simmering. Poach until fish are completely opaque and tender – about 8 minutes. Plate fish and ladle broth over fish.
Serves 4. 275 Calories per serving.

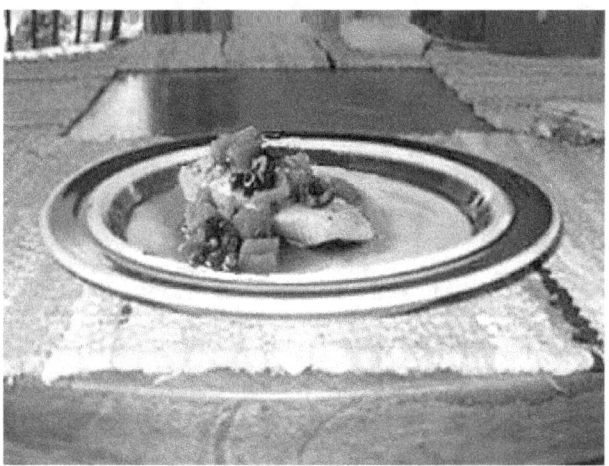

Diet Tip of the Day: **A good reducing diet must help you remain healthy** while you are losing weight.

Recipe 36

<u>Chicken Piccata</u>

  1 pound boneless skinless chicken breast halves
  2 teaspoons olive oil
  1 teaspoon minced garlic
  ¼ cup shallots, diced
  ¾ pound fresh green beans, washed and snipped
  1 teaspoon lemon juice
  ¼ cup capers, rinsed
  2 fresh lemons, cut into small wedges

In a skillet, heat olive oil and minced garlic over medium heat. Sauté chicken breasts and shallots for two to three minutes, tossing often, until chicken is partially cooked. Add green beans and one teaspoon of lemon juice and sauté for an additional two to three minutes, or until chicken is completely cooked and green beans are al dente. Add capers; and cover chicken. Let sit for one more minute to warm capers. Serve immediately with wedges of lemon.
<u>Serves 4</u>. 270 calories per serving

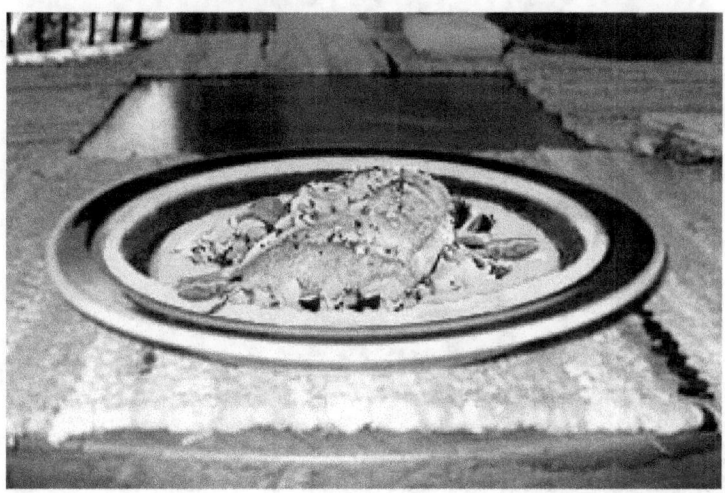

<u>Diet Tip of the Day:</u> Handle **occasional overeating by compensating**. To do this, estimate how far you have strayed from your weight-loss diet and then make amends at the next opportunity (usually the next meal or two) – by eating less.

Recipe 37

Beans & Greens Salad

⅓ cup chopped oregano
⅓ cup chopped parsley
3 cloves garlic, chopped
1 lemon, juiced

Prepare dressing by combining above ingredients and stirring in ¼ cup extra-virgin olive oil. Salt and pepper to taste.

½ pound mesclun mix
¼ pound green beans
19-ounce can garbanzo beans (chickpeas)

Arrange mesclun mix, garbanzo beans and green beans on a large platter. Drizzle dressing over beans and greens.
Serves 4. Approximately 260 Calories per serving.

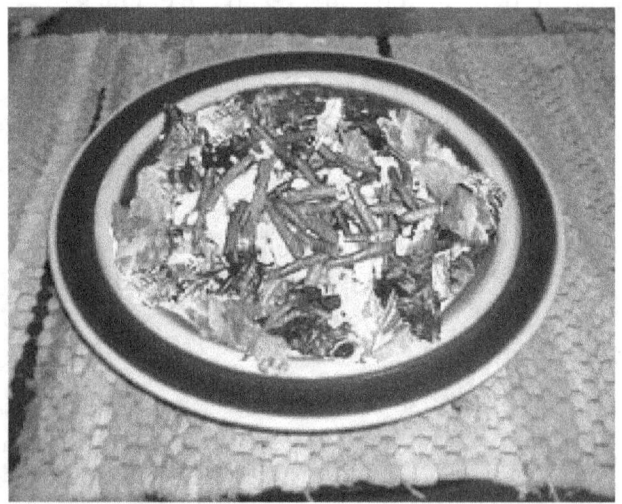

Diet Tip of the Day: Fat-free isn't always your best bet. Low fat doesn't necessarily mean low calorie! Most often sugar is substituted for fat and the calorie total remains the same or even higher. Instead, look for low-calorie or reduced-calorie foods.

Recipe 38

Pan-Fried Sole

  4   sole fillets (6-ounces each), skinned
  1   tablespoon olive oil

Salsa Ingredients:
  1 pint cherry tomatoes, quartered
  ¾ cup cucumber, finely chopped
  ⅓ cup yellow bell pepper, finely chopped
  3 tablespoons fresh basil, chopped
  2 tablespoons capers
  1½ tablespoons shallots, finely chopped
  1 tablespoon balsamic vinegar
  2 teaspoons lemon rind, grated

Combine salsa ingredients in a bowl and stir in ½ teaspoon salt and ⅛
teaspoon black pepper. Mix thoroughly.

Heat olive oil in a large nonstick skillet over medium-high heat. Season sole
fillets with
½ teaspoon salt and ⅛ teaspoon black pepper. Add fish to pan; cook about
1½ minutes on each side or until fish flakes easily when tested with a fork.
Spoon salsa over fish and serve immediately.

Serves 4. 325 Calories per serving

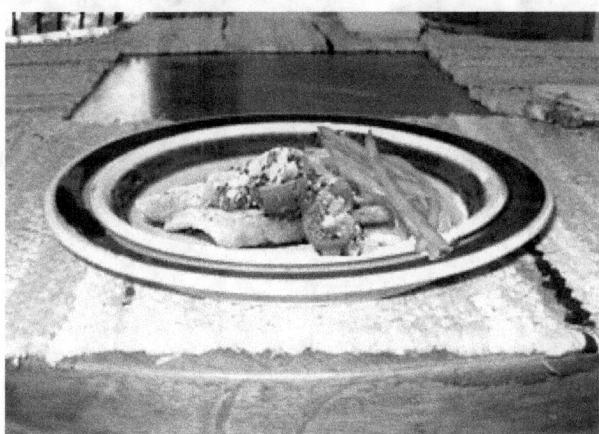

Diet Tip of the Day: If you are overweight start on a weight loss diet now
because it will only become **more difficult to lose weight as you get older**.

Recipe 39

Beef Steak Strips

　　1 lb top loin sirloin, or top round about ¾" thick
　　1 tsp garlic, finely chopped
　　½ tsp dry thyme
　　½ tsp salt and ¼ tsp black peppercorns

Cut the steak into 3-inch long by ¼-inch thick strips Sprinkle the beef strips with garlic, thyme, salt and pepper. Prepare a large non-stick skillet over medium-high heat. Add the steak strips and shake the skillet constantly to avoid sticking. Cook approximately 2 to 3 minutes until meat is seared but pink inside. Check the center by making small incision.
Serves 4. About 330 Calories per serving (meat only).

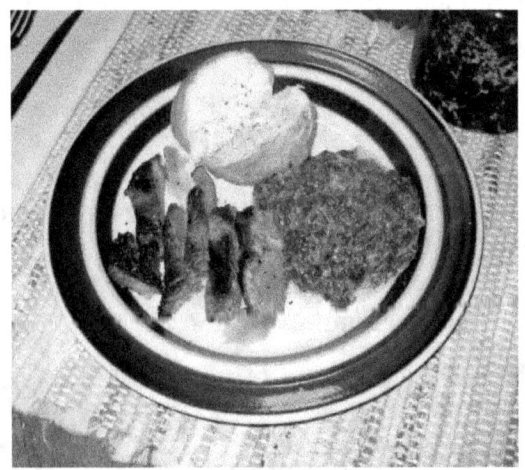

Diet Tip of the Day: Bear in mind, that knowledge and the discipline to **workout regularly** are far more important than fancy equipment.

Recipe 40

Grilled Scallops &Polenta

1 pound sea scallops
¾ cup polenta cornmeal
¾ cup skim milk
1 medium Portobello mushroom
½ pound green beans
¼ cup chopped red onion
16 asparagus spear
1 teaspoon extra-virgin olive oil

Bring 1½ cups of water and skim milk to rapid boil. Add salt to taste and slowly add polenta while stirring. Reduce heat. Continue stirring until desired consistency is reached. Pour polenta into lightly greased pan. After polenta has cooled cover and refrigerate. Cut chilled polenta into 4 pieces. Grill on medium-hot fire – about two minutes on each side.

Brush Portobello mushroom and asparagus spear with olive oil and place on grill for about 3 minutes on each side.

Grill scallops on medium-hot fire. Turn after two minutes or when first side turns opaque. Grill until second side turns opaque – about another 2 minutes. Don't overcook but test a scallop by cutting to make sure it's cooked through. Salt and pepper to taste.

Serves 4. The food on the plate pictured below totals about 380 Calories.

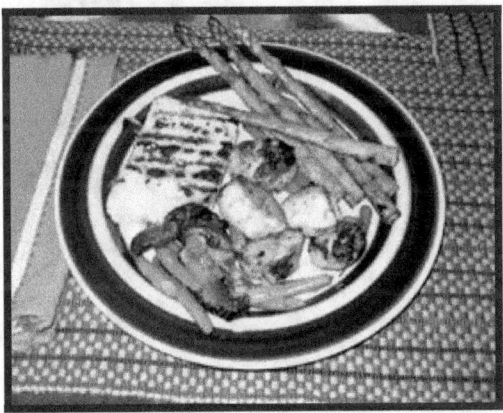

Diet Tip of the Day: To have better control of what you eat **bring your lunch to work**.

Pork Chop with Orange Slices

4	loin pork chops, ½-inch-thick (about 1½ lbs total, including bones)
8	orange slices, ¼-inch-thick
1	teaspoon salt
¾	teaspoon black pepper
¼	cup orange marmalade preserve
½	cup bottled fruit-based barbecue sauce

such as Grandville's Gourmet BBQ Sauce

Marinade: ½ cup orange juice, 2 teaspoons soy sauce and ¼ teaspoon crushed red pepper.

Combine pork chops and marinade in large re-sealable plastic bag. Refrigerate for about 30 minutes. Remove chops from marinade and season with salt and black pepper.

Stir together orange marmalade and BBQ sauce in a small bowl. Brush one side of pork chops evenly with half of marmalade-BBQ mixture. Grill chops, with marmalade-BBQ mixture side up over medium-high heat (about 375°) for about 5 minutes or until done. Turn chops, and brush with remaining marmalade-BBQ mixture. Grill another 5 minutes or until done. Grill orange slices over medium-high heat, 1 minute on each side.

Serves 4. 470 Calories per serving (includes pork chop and two orange slices).

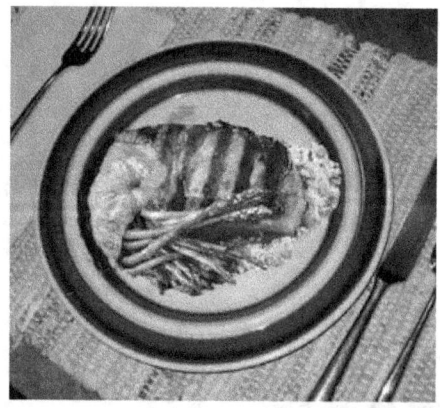

Diet Tip of the Day: Make sure fat is trimmed from meat. Most meats are about 80 Calories per ounce – whereas, pure fat is 256 Calories per ounce!

Recipe 42a

<u>Low-Cal Smoothie</u>

Smoothies are delicious, nutritious and fun to drink! They're great for a fast but nutritious breakfast, a light energy-boosting lunch, a healthy snack, a late afternoon pick me up, and a delicious dessert. Making your own smoothie is a smart way to save money and get healthy at the same time!

    8 ounces plain fat-free yogurt
    1 cup orange juice
    1 cup strawberries
    ½ cup blueberries
    1 banana
    1 teaspoon sugar
    1 teaspoon vanilla extract

Place yogurt, strawberries, and blueberries in a blender. Pour in orange juice. Add sugar and vanilla extract to mixture. Blend all ingredients until thick and smooth. Pour smoothie into a glass and enjoy.

<u>Serves 2</u>. About 220 Calories per serving

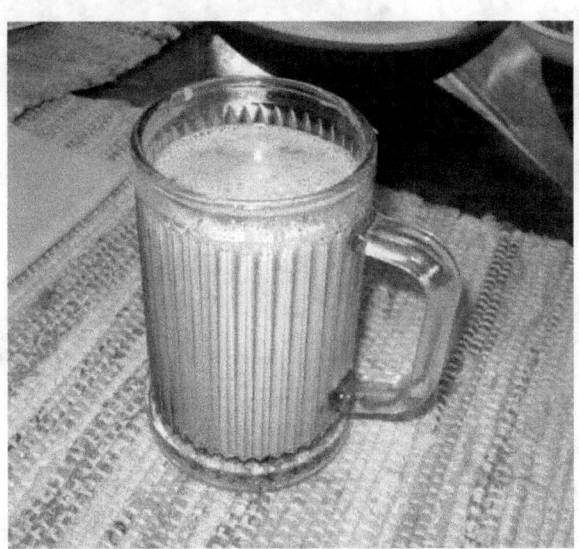

<u>Diet Tip of the Day:</u> Two scientific journals indicate **dark chocolate** - not white chocolate or milk chocolate - is potent antioxidant and is good for you. But don't overdo it, because you have to offset the extra chocolate calories by eating less of other foods.

Recipe 42b

Healthy Pasta Salad

½   pound fusilli pasta, cooked until tender but firm
2   broccoli crowns, chopped
¼   pint cherry tomatoes (about 8), halved
½   cup black olives, halved
½   cup garbanzo beans (chick peas)
½   cup fresh "light" mozzarella, chopped
1   tablespoon basil
1   tablespoon rosemary
2   teaspoons garlic powder
¼   cup of a **recommended dressing** (page 10)

Combine dry ingredients in a medium-size bowl. Stir in salad dressing. Mix thoroughly. Salt and black pepper to taste.
Serves 4. 370 Calories per serving.

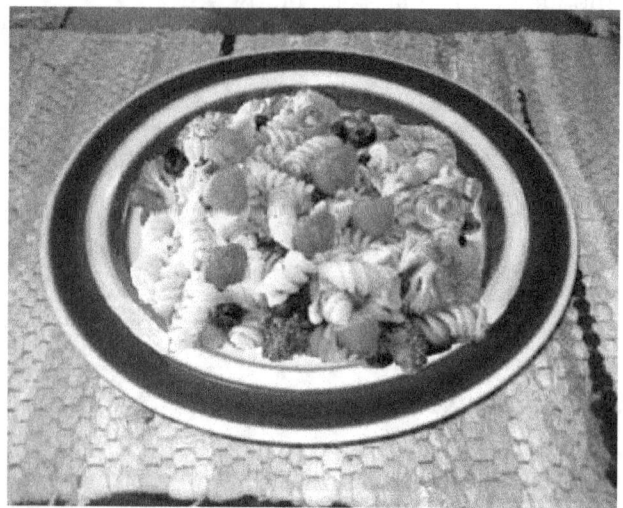

Diet Tip of the Day: Ask yourself: **"Why am I overweight**?"   Do you eat too much of everything? Too much dessert? Drink too much beer? Is your only exercise walking from the TV to the refrigerator? Determine the why and then focus on one or two of your problem areas. Sometimes it's that simple.

Recipe 43

<u>Beef Burgundy</u>

  1 lb boneless beef chuck, trimmed & cut in 1" pieces
  2 large carrots, cut into 1-inch pieces
  1 medium onion, cut into 1-inch pieces
  1 tablespoon flour
  1 tablespoon tomato paste
  1 clove garlic, crushed
  1 tablespoon olive oil
  1 cup dry red wine
  2 sprigs fresh thyme
  10 ounces mushrooms, sliced in half
  8 ounces frozen peas

In Dutch oven, heat oil on medium-high until hot. Add beef and cook 5 to 6 minutes or until beef is browned on all sides. Transfer beef to a bowl. Preheat oven to 325° F. To drippings in Dutch oven, add carrots, garlic, and onion. Stir occasionally. Cook 10 minutes or until vegetables are browned and tender. Stir in flour, tomato paste, ½ teaspoon salt, and ¼ teaspoon black pepper, and cook another minute. Add wine and heat to boiling, stirring until browned bits from bottom of Dutch oven are loosened. Return meat and juice in the bowl to Dutch oven. Add thyme and mushrooms; bring to a boil. Cover and bake 1½ hours or until meat is fork-tender. Discard thyme sprigs. Before stew is done, cook peas per package instructions. Then add peas to Dutch oven.
<u>Serves 4</u>. 350 Calories per serving

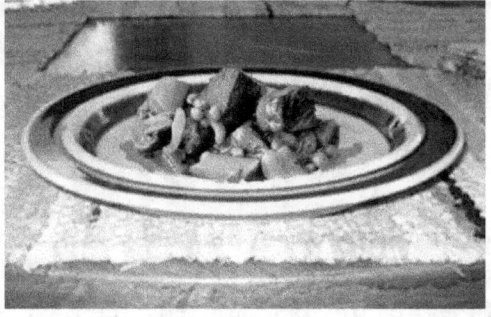

<u>Diet Tip of the Day:</u> When on a diet **simple is better**. Why? Because simple, uncomplicated meals usually contain fewer "hidden calories" than more elaborate dishes.

Recipe 44

<u>Chicken Cutlet</u>

Buy 4 skinless, boneless chicken cutlets or breast halves (about 1 lb), flattened to about ¼ to ½-inch thick.

- ¾ cup Panko bread crumbs
- ⅓ cup grated Parmesan cheese
- 1 egg, beaten
- 4 tablespoons extra-virgin olive oil, divided

Season chicken cutlets with salt and pepper. Combine bread crumbs and Parmesan cheese in a shallow bowl. Whisk egg in a separate shallow bowl. Dip chicken in egg and then coat both sides in crumb mixture.

Heat 2 tablespoons of olive oil in large skillet over medium-high heat. Add 2 cutlets, and cook 2 minutes on each side or until cooked through. Repeat with 2 tablespoons olive oil and remaining 2 cutlets. Serve hot.

<u>Serves 4</u>. 450 Calories per serving (chicken cutlet only)

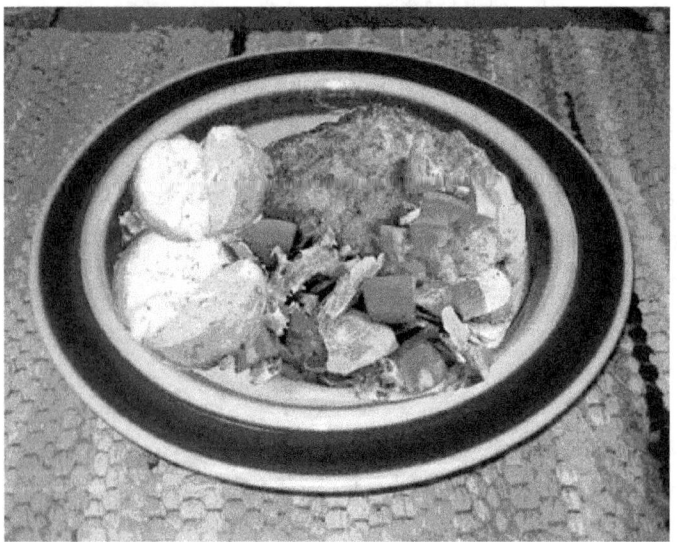

<u>Diet Tip of the Day</u>: **Working out at home** has some significant advantages. Your workout takes less time because you don't have to drive back and forth to a fitness facility; and you have the flexibility of dividing your workout into small time segments to fit your day, and working out at home is less expensive.

Recipe 45

Personal-Size Meat Loaf

- 1 pound extra lean ground beef
- ⅓ cup quick oats
- 2 egg whites
- ½ cup chipotle salsa, divided
- ¼ cup ketchup, divided

Place egg whites in a large bowl, mixing well with a whisk. Stir in oats, 6 tablespoons salsa, and 2 tablespoons ketchup. Add beef and mix well. Divide beef mixture into 4 equal portions, shaping each into an oval-shaped loaf. and place loaves on baking pan lined with tin foil and coated with cooking spray. Bake in preheated oven at 350°F for 30 minutes or until done.

Combine remaining 2 tablespoons salsa and 2 tablespoons ketchup in a small bowl. Spread mixture evenly over individual meat loaves.

Serves 4. 410 Calories per serving (meat loaf only)

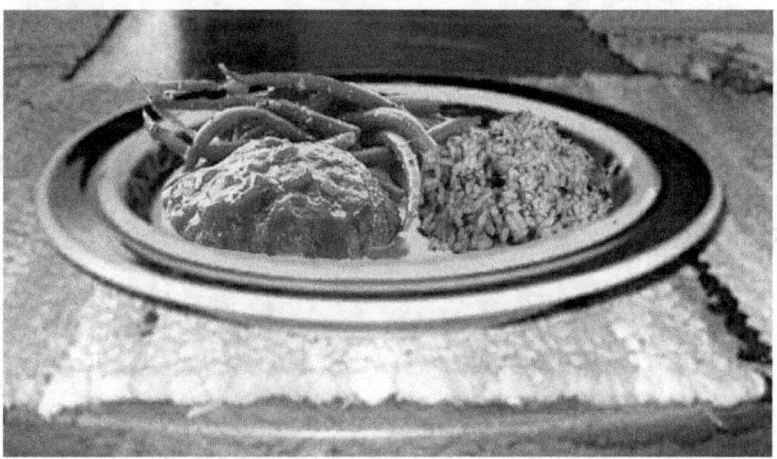

Diet Tip of the Day: To make sure you stay on track, **weigh in once a week**. There may be times when you might not see a weight loss, often because lost fat is temporarily replaced by water. This condition will gradually be corrected as you continue dieting.

Recipe 46

Crab Cakes

- 1 lb jumbo crab meat
- 1½ Tbsp light mayonnaise
- 1½ Tbsp chopped green bell pepper
- 2 medium green onions, chopped
- 1 large egg, beaten
- 1 cup panko bread crumbs
- 2 Tbsp canola oil
- ¼ tsp black pepper

Drain crab meat on layers of paper towels. Combine crab meat, bell pepper, mayonnaise, black pepper, onions and egg. Stir in ¼ cup panko bread crumbs. (Place remaining panko in shallow dish.)

Divide crab meat mixture into 8 portions. Shape portions into ¾-inch thick patties and dredge in panko. Place non-stick skillet over medium heat and add 1 Tbsp oil. Add dredged patties and cook 3 minutes on each side or until golden.

Prepare remoulade: Combine ¼ cup light mayonnaise, 2 tsp minced shallots, 1 tsp chopped tarragon, 1 tsp chopped parsley, 1½ tsp Dijon mustard and ¾ tsp wine vinegar. Serve remoulade with crab cakes.
Serves 4. 320 Calories per serving (2 crab cakes)

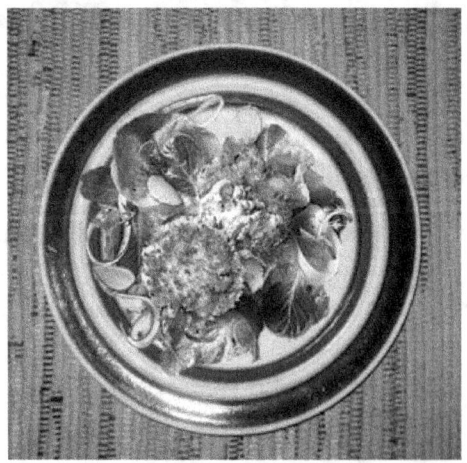

Recipe 47

Black-Eyed Peas over Rice

2 cups fat-free, lower-sodium chicken broth
2 slices smoked bacon
2 cups water
½ teaspoon kosher salt
½ teaspoon freshly ground black pepper
1-pound bag frozen black-eyed peas, thawed
12-ounce bunch fresh turnip greens, trimmed and coarsely chopped
2 tablespoons pepper vinegar

Cook bacon in a Dutch oven over medium heat until crisp. Remove bacon from pan using a slotted spoon, reserving drippings in pan. Crumble bacon.

Add onion to drippings in pan; sauté 4 minutes, stirring occasionally. Stir in broth and the next 5 ingredients (through greens); bring to a boil. Reduce heat, and simmer for about an hour or until peas are tender, stirring occasionally and skimming as necessary. Stir in vinegar. Ladle about 1⅓ cups pea mixture into each of 4 bowls and top evenly with crumbled bacon. **Serves 4**. 280 Calories per serving (does not include rice)

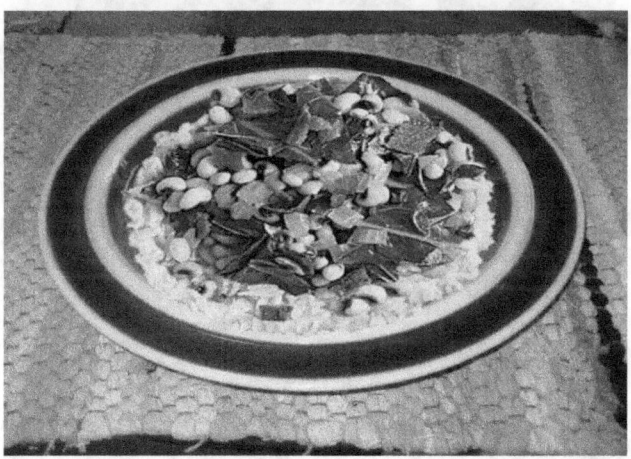

Two servings of black-eyed peas over brown rice on platter.

Diet Tip of the Day: Black-eyed peas are a wonderful food but **black-eyed peas are an incomplete protein**. If however black-eyed peas are eaten with a grain such as rice, the combination forms a complete protein – just as complete a protein as meat, poultry, or fish!

164

Recipe 48

Pasta Pomodoro

Pasta Pomodoro (Italian for pasta with tomatoes) is typically prepared with angel hair pasta, olive oil, fresh tomatoes, and fresh basil. It's light, delicious and easy to make.

- ¾ pound angel hair pasta
- 1½ pints cherry tomatoes (about 45), halved
- 8 fresh basil leaves, chopped
- 4 cloves garlic, minced
- 2 tablespoons olive oil
- 4 Tbsp grated parmesan cheese

Cook angel hair pasta per package directions. Over medium heat, sauté the garlic in olive oil until it just starts to turn golden. Add tomatoes and cook for about 10 minutes, or until they just start to release juices. Turn off the heat and stir basil into the sauce. Over the cooked pasta, spoon the tomato sauce with a little of the pasta water and garnish with more basil and grated cheese. **Serves 4**. 420 Calories per serving

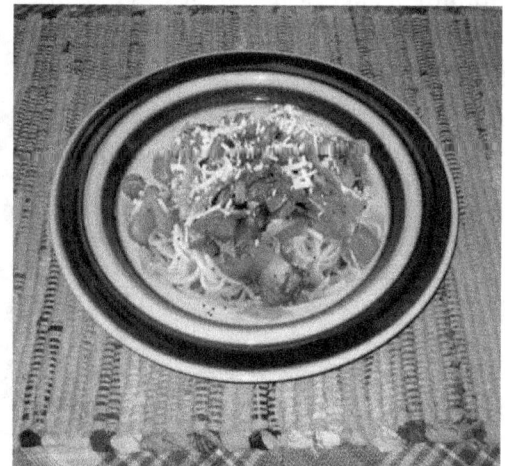

Above prepared with mix of cherry and plum tomatoes.

Diet Tip of the Day: Thinking about using **honey** rather than sugar? Honey has about 21 calories per teaspoon while sugar has 15. And the vitamin and mineral content of honey is very low.

Recipe 49

Healthy Frittata

3 large eggs, plus 3 egg whites
¾ cup reduced-fat cottage cheese
4 ounces smoked gouda cheese, shredded (about 1 cup)
1 teaspoon minced fresh rosemary
3 cloves garlic, thinly sliced
2 tablespoons EVOO
1 medium onion, chopped
16-ounce package frozen mixed vegetables, thawed
2 tablespoons grated parmesan cheese
1 scant teaspoon paprika

1) Position a rack in the upper third of your oven and preheat to 450 degrees F. Whisk eggs and egg whites in a bowl. Add the cottage cheese and whisk until almost smooth. Whisk in the gouda and rosemary. In a 10-inch nonstick skillet over medium-high, cook the garlic in the olive oil. Heat until garlic starts to brown, about 1 to 2 minutes. Add onion, season with salt and cook 2 minutes. Add the vegetables, increase the heat to high and cook until just tender, about 5 minutes. Reduce the heat to medium.

2) Spread the egg mixture evenly in the pan. Cook, without disturbing until a thin crust forms on the bottom, about 2 minutes. Run a rubber spatula around the edge to release egg from the pan. Continue cooking until the bottom is golden, about 2 to 3 minutes. Sprinkle with the parmesan and paprika. Transfer skillet to the oven and bake about 5 to 7 minutes. Remove from the oven, cover and let sit, 5 to 7 minutes. Cut into 4 wedges.
Serves 4. 320 Calories per serving (¼ of frittata)

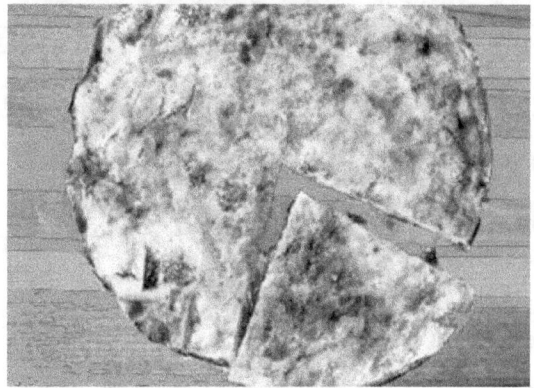

Photo shows frittata on cutting board - hot from skillet.

Recipe 50

Mediterranean Chicken

    4 small boneless skinless chicken breasts (about 1 lb total)
    1 tablespoon paprika
    1 tablespoon olive oil
    ½ teaspoon snipped fresh rosemary
    2 cloves garlic, minced
    ¼ teaspoon ground black pepper
    ¼ cup dry red wine
    3 tablespoons balsamic vinegar

Place chicken breast halves between two pieces of plastic wrap and pound with the flat side of a meat mallet into a rectangle ¼ to ½ inch thick. In a small bowl, combine paprika, oil, rosemary, garlic, and pepper; mixing well until it becomes a paste. Rub both sides of each chicken breast with paste mixture. Coat a 13x9x2-inch baking pan with nonstick cooking spray. Place coated chicken in prepared pan; cover and refrigerate for 2 to 6 hours.

Preheat oven to 450ºF. Drizzle chicken with wine. Bake for 6 to 8 minutes or until the chicken is no longer pink and a meat thermometer inserted in the thickest portion of the chicken registers 170ºF and the juices run clear. Turn the chicken once halfway through baking.

Remove from oven. Immediately drizzle vinegar onto chicken in the baking pan. Transfer chicken to serving plates. Stir the liquid in the baking pan and drizzle over chicken. If desired, garnish with fresh rosemary.
Serves 4. 180 Calories per serving (not including spaghetti squash & green beans).

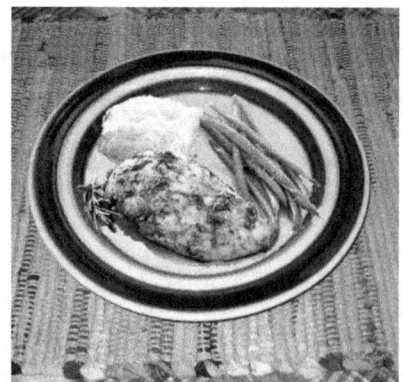

Photo shows chicken with spaghetti squash & green beans.

Appendix A
Shopping Tips

No cooking doesn't mean no preparation! You will probably have to shop once a week. The following should help you prepare your shopping list.

First, understand that the problem with basing a meal plan on name-brand food items, such as a particular Lean Cuisine frozen entree, is that the item might not be available where you shop, or it may have been discontinued. What to do? That's where Appendices C and D in this book come in handy. Appendix C lists 19 name-brand soups in microwaveable bowls. Appendix D lists more than 100 name-brand frozen meals with their calorie count. Using these lists you should be able to find a substitute for the soup or frozen entree you can't find - a substitute that is based on the same food type, e.g., chicken, fish, or meat, and has the same approximate calorie count.

Substituting Foods

If there is a food listed in the diet you don't like, or perhaps that you forgot to pick up while shopping, you probably can exchange or substitute another food in its place – a technique used by dieticians. Exchanging a food listed in a diet for another food with approximately equal caloric value and nutritional content is the foundation of a successful long-term diet.

Substitution possibilities are almost endless but have to be done carefully. The easiest substitutions are those within the same food group, such as exchanging one vegetable variety for another, or a glass of milk for a cup of yogurt. More sophisticated exchanges cross food groups, for instance replacing 3½ ounces of turkey with a tablespoon of peanut butter spread on a piece of whole wheat bread. Both foods are complete proteins and both contain about 175 Calories. Refer to a good online calorie table to find calorie values. With some understanding and experience, you will be able to substitute foods called for in this diet with equal calorie foods from the same food group.

If there is a food listed in the *50-Day Flex Diet* that you don't like, or perhaps that you forgot to pick up while shopping, you probably can exchange or substitute another food in its place – a technique used by dieticians. Exchanging a food listed in a diet for another food with approximately equal caloric value and nutritional content is the foundation of many successful long-term diets. Substitution possibilities are almost endless but have to be done carefully. The easiest substitutions are those within the same food group, such as exchanging one vegetable variety for another, or a glass of milk for a cup of yogurt. More sophisticated exchanges cross food groups, such as replacing 3½ ounces of turkey with a tablespoon of peanut butter on a piece of whole-grain bread. Both foods are complete protein and both contain about 175 Calories. With some understanding and experience, you can use this table to help you substitute foods called for in the *50-Day Flex Diet* with equal calorie foods from the same food group.

Breakfast: You may substitute any cereal for any other wholesome cereal. For example, if you're not crazy about having Shredded Wheat for breakfast on Day 6, substitute Wheat Chex or Cheerios, etc. But remember to adjust the amount of cereal to account for the calorie difference between brands. If you don't like the soft-boiled egg called for on Day 9, cook a fried egg instead. And if Cantaloupe is on the menu but is not in season, replace cantaloupe with a half cup of orange juice – both contain about 50 Calories.

Snacks: Again, where yogurt is specified you may substitute an 6-ounce glass of skim milk, but to maintain a nutritionally balanced diet keep this snack a dairy selection. Similarly, when fruit is on the agenda, you may select any type of fruit but do not stray from the fruit group. Nuts and popcorn can be interchanged at will. Specified convenient brand-name snacks, such as Skinny Cow ice cream, Kashi Granola bars, Nabisco 100 Calorie Pack cookies and Orville Redenbacher's Smart Pop Popcorn should be widely available but other equivalent brands may be substituted if need be. Just make sure the substitute snack has a calorie count that is the same, or very close, to the specified snack.

Another alternative is the following Food Substitution List that suggests substitutions for a variety of food items that appear in the daily meal plans. For example, Day 5 of the diet calls for half a cantaloupe for breakfast. But suppose cantaloupe is not in season, or just doesn't look good, or maybe it's too expensive, or you can't find it at your grocery, from the Food Substitution List you find that you may exchange a ½ cup of orange juice for half cantaloupe – both are in the fruit category and both contain about 50 Calories.

Light Syrup - Use any light syrup (25 Calories per Tbsp)
Big-Bowl Salad - Exchange with unlimited steamed greens (spinach, etc)
Cantaloupe (½) - Use ½ cup Orange juice
Cereal - Exchange with any other whole-grain cereal
Cottage Cheese (1 cup) - Two 8 oz glasses skim milk
Yogurt - Select 6 ounces skim milk
Eggs – Use Egg Beaters
Fresh fruit - ¾ cup canned fruit (no sugar added)

Frozen entrée - Substitute frozen entrée with same calories.
Grapefruit (½) - Choose an orange (medium)
Handful of Nuts - Popcorn Mini Bag
Kashi Chewy Granola Bar - Quaker Chewy Dipps Granola Bar
Kashi Go Lean Waffles - Eggo Nutri-Grain Whole Wheat Frozen Waffles
Hot Pockets Wraps - Lean Pockets Wraps
Morningstar Breakfast Sausage - Any breakfast sausage with comparable calories
String Cheese - Laughing Cow light cheese (2 wedges)
Popcorn - Use handful of mixed nuts
Raisin bread - Plain whole-grain bread
Skinny Cow Ice Cream Sandwich - Skinny Cow Fudge Ice Cream Bar
Soup - Choose any soup with same calorie count
Whole-grain Bread - Vary bread type (whole wheat, rye, etc)
Wine (4 oz) - Instead select grapes (1 cup)

Shopping Tip: The danger of basing a meal plan on name brand food items, such as frozen entrees, is that the item may not be available where you shop, or it may have been discontinued. What to do? That's where Appendices B, and D, in this book come in handy. **Appendix B** (on the following page) lists 19 name-brand soups in microwaveable bowls. **Appendix D** (on pages 174 to 179) lists nearly 150 name-brand frozen entrees. Using these lists you should be able to find a substitute for the food you can't find, a substitute that is based on the same food type, e.g., chicken, fish, or meat, and has the same approximate calorie count. So, **if you cannot find the exact item called for in the diet (because it's out of stock or discontinued), substitute a comparable food (of the same type with about the same caloric value).**

In summary, remember that whenever you encounter a product on this diet, such as "Skinny Cow Ice Cream Sandwich" or "Kashi Go Lean Waffles," that has been discontinued or is out of stock, substitute an equivalent food or desert that is of approximately equal caloric value and nutritional content. In other words substitute a different ice cream product for the "Skinny Cow Ice Cream Sandwich" or a another waffle brand for the "Kashi Go Lean Waffles."

Appendix B
Soup Selections

When the Daily Meal Plan menu specifies soup have only one serving (8 ounces) unless stated otherwise. Note that the listed soups were available in most supermarkets as of 07/21/2020. *These are a canned soup selections.

Soup Description	Calories
Healthy Choice Chicken with Rice	90
Campbell's Tomato	100
Healthy Choice Country Vegetable	100
Progresso Minestrone*	110
Progresso Chickarina*	110
Progresso Italian-Style Wedding*	120
Campbell's Home-Style Light Chicken Corn Chowder*	120
Campbell's Home-Style Chicken Noodle	130
Campbell's Home-Style Butter Nut Squash*	130
Campbell's Healthy Request Vegetable Beef	140
Progresso Lentil*	140
Progresso Green Split Pea*	150
Campbell's Slow Kettle New England Clam Chowder	160
Progresso Macaroni and Bean*	160
Progresso New England Clam Chowder*	170
Progresso Lasagna-Style*	170
Progresso Broccoli Cheese with Bacon*	180
As an alternative, have 2 servings of a 90 Calorie soup	180
Campbell's Chunky Classic Chicken Noodle	190
Amy's Rustic Italian Vegetable*	190
Campbell's Chunky Beef n Cheese*	200
Amy's French Country Vegetable*	210
Campbell's Chunky Sirloin Burger + Vegetables	220
Enjoy two servings of a 110 or 120 Calorie soup	230
Enjoy two servings of a 120 Calorie soup	240

Appendix C
Important Frozen Food Information

Busy families, singles, older people, and office workers alike enjoy the simplicity and convenience of a frozen meal. Many offices have an employee freezer jammed with all kinds frozen meals, which get zapped in a microwave for a quick, portable, portion-controlled, and relatively inexpensive lunch.

In some cases, frozen may actually be better than fresh, because if you keep fresh fruit and vegetables your fridge for a long time, they lose some of their nutritional value. Whereas, frozen foods are usually processed and packaged within hours of being picked. And the freezing process itself does not destroy nutrients. So buying frozen and then defrosting when you want the fruit or vegetable can actually retain more nutrients.

Storing Frozen Foods
According to the U.S. Department of Agriculture, food stored continuously at 0°F is always safe to eat. Freezing keeps food safe and preserves food for extended periods because it prevents the growth of microorganisms that cause both food spoilage and food-borne illness.

Use an appliance thermometer to monitor your freezer's temperature. If a refrigerator freezing compartment can't maintain 0 °F or if the freezer door is opened frequently, use it for short-term food storage, and eat those foods as soon as possible for best quality. Use a free-standing freezer set at 0 °F or below for long-term storage of frozen foods. Again, keep a thermometer in your freezing compartment or freezer to check the temperature.

Because freezing keeps food safe almost indefinitely, recommended freezer storage times are to preserve quality (taste, etc) of food, not the safety or nutritional value. **The quality of frozen dinners or entrees in a freezer at 0 °F will be maintained for 3 to 4 months**.

If there is a power outage, or if your freezer fails, or if the freezer door is left ajar by mistake, the food may still be safe to use. As long as a freezer with its door ajar continues to run, to cool, the foods should stay safe overnight. If a repairman is on the way or it appears the power will be restored soon, just keep your freezer door closed. A freezer full of food will usually keep about 2 days if the door is kept shut; a half-full freezer will last about a day. The freezing compartment of a refrigerator may not keep foods frozen as long. If the freezer is not full, group packages together to help maintain their low temperature.

During a power failure, you may want to put dry ice, a block or bags of ice in the freezer, or transfer foods to a friend's freezer until power returns. Again, use an appliance thermometer to monitor the temperature. To determine the safety of foods when the power goes on, check their condition and temperature. If food is partly frozen, still has ice crystals, or is as cold as if it were in a refrigerator (40 °F), it is safe to refreeze or use. It's not necessary to cook raw foods before refreezing. **If in doubt discard the food. And always discard frozen food whose temperature has exceeded 40 °F for more than two hours.**

Frozen Food Safety

Increasingly, food giants like ConAgra, Nestlé and others that supply Americans with processed foods concede that they cannot ensure the safety of their food products. Frozen foods pose a particularly serious safety problem because unsuspecting consumers buy frozen foods for their convenience and incorrectly believe that cooking frozen foods is a matter of taste – not safety.

Still the food industry says that extensive outbreaks of food-borne illness are rare, even though it is well-known that most of the millions of cases of food-borne illness every year go unreported or are not traced to the source. For example, each year approximately 40,000 cases of salmonella poisoning are reported in the United States – but perhaps as many as one million cases go unreported. (Salmonella is a type of bacteria most often found in poultry, eggs, unprocessed milk, meat and water.) Recently salmonella pathogens in some frozen meals have sickened thousands of people.

How could this happen? First, the supply chain for ingredients in processed foods – from flour to fruits and vegetables to flavorings – is becoming more complex and global in the drive to keep food costs down. As a result, government and industry officials concede that almost every food ingredient is now a potential carrier of pathogens. A further complication is that a large number of food companies subcontract processing work to save money and don't require suppliers to test for pathogens. In fact, companies often don't even know who is supplying their ingredients.

In addition, many frozen-food manufacturers have stopped cooking their products at high temperatures, a tactic they call the "kill step," which is intended to eliminate any lingering microbes. Frequently this process step turns some of the frozen food ingredients into mush. So, instead the "kill step" has been shifted to consumers. For example, ConAgra has added food safety instructions to its frozen meals, including the Healthy Choice brand. A

173

typical "frozen-food safety" instruction offers this guidance: "Internal temperature needs to reach 165°F as measured by a food thermometer in several spots." General Mills, now advises consumers to avoid microwaves altogether and cook their frozen pizzas only in a conventional oven.

Bottom line: To be safe, always cook frozen foods so that the internal temperature reaches 165°F as measured by a good food thermometer.

The Sodium Problem

Sodium and sodium chloride (salt) normally occur in small quantities in many natural foods. People also add salt during food preparation and to the food they eat. But the average sodium intake for American adults is about 3,400 mg daily – more than 1,000 mg higher than the upper limit of 2,400 mg per day recommended by the U.S. Department of Health and Human Services and the Department of Agriculture Dietary Guidelines. (Note that one level teaspoon of salt contains about 2,300 mg of sodium.)

Although sodium plays an important role in your body, many studies have demonstrated that high sodium intake results in excessive water retention which causes blood volume to expand which in turn raises blood pressure. Moreover, some people are more sensitive to the effects of sodium than are others. These sodium-sensitive people retain sodium more easily. If you're in that group, extra sodium in your diet increases your chance of developing high blood pressure, a condition that can lead to cardiovascular and kidney diseases. Individuals who have high blood pressure and who are also salt sensitive are frequently advised to limit their sodium intake even further.

The downside to commercially prepared frozen entrees is that they frequently are loaded with too much salt (sodium). Be aware that, because of the relatively high sodium content of the frozen dinners and microwaveable soups, **the *90-Day No-Cooking Diet* may not be appropriate for everyone.**

In fact, you should have a medical checkup before beginning this weight loss diet. And you should let your physician know that the *90-Day No-Cooking Diet* relies to a large degree on commercially processed convenience foods (frozen and microwaveable) – many of which have a relatively high salt (sodium) content.

Appendix D: Frozen Entrees

Appendix D lists three popular brands of frozen entrées: Healthy Choice, Lean Cuisine and Smart Ones. The listing is further divided by entrée type: Poultry entrées, Meat entrées, Seafood entrées, Pasta entrées, Pizza and Other entrées. The entire table is arranged from the lowest to highest in calories. Note that the listed frozen entrées were available in most super markets as of 07/21/2020.

Entrée Type	Name	Brand	Calories
Poultry	Tomato Basil Chicken & Spinach	Smart Ones	160
Meat	Steak Portobella	Lean Cuisine	160
Meat	Asian Style Beef & Broccoli	Smart Ones	~~160~~ 170
Poultry	Herb Roasted Chicken	Lean Cuisine	170
Poultry	Slow Roasted Turkey Breast	Smart Ones	170
Poultry	Grilled Chicken Marsala	Healthy Choice	180
Poultry	Creamy Basil Chicken w Broccoli	Smart Ones	~~180~~ 170
Poultry	Garlic Chicken Rolls	Lean Cuisine	180
Meat	Beef Merlot	Healthy Choice	180
Meat	Homestyle Beef Pot Roast	Smart Ones	180
Poultry	Roasted Turkey & Vegetables	Lean Cuisine	190
Poultry	Chicken & Broccoli Alfredo	Healthy Choice	190
Poultry	Chicken & Vegetable Stir Fry	Healthy Choice	190
Other	Broccoli & Cheddar Roast Potato	Smart Ones	190
Poultry	Crustless Chicken Pot Pie	Smart Ones	~~200~~ 190
Poultry	Buffalo Style Chicken	Lean Cuisine	~~200~~ 190
Poultry	Home Style Chicken & Potatoes	Healthy Choice	200
Pasta	Angel Hair Marinara	Smart Ones	200
Poultry	Salisbury Steak	Smart Ones	200
Meat	Roast Beef & Mashed Potatoes	Smart Ones	~~220~~ 200
Pasta	Primavera Pasta	Smart Ones	210
Poultry	Honey Balsamic Chicken	Healthy Choice	210

Entrée Type	Name	Brand	Calories
Pasta	Ravioli Florentine	Smart Ones	210
Poultry	Cajun Style Chicken & Shrimp	Healthy Choice	220
Pasta	Cheese Ravioli Mushroom Sauce	Smart Ones	230
Poultry	Ranchero Chicken Wrap	Smart Ones	230
Poultry	Lemon Herb Chicken Picante	Smart Ones	230
Pasta	Cheese Ravioli Mushroom Sauce	Smart Ones	230
Meat	Meat Loaf with Mashed Potatoes	Lean Cuisine	~~230~~ 240
Seafood	Shrimp Alfredo	Lean Cuisine	~~230~~ 240
Poultry	Chicken Margherita	Smart Ones	~~220~~ 240
Poultry	Grilled Chicken Caesar	Lean Cuisine	240
Poultry	Honey Glazed Turkey & Potatoes	Healthy Choice	240
Pasta	Spicy Penne Arrabbiata	Lean Cuisine	240
Pasta	Four Cheese Cannelloni	Lean Cuisine	~~240~~ 250
Poultry	Creamy Basil Chicken w Tortellini	Lean Cuisine	~~240~~ 250
Pasta	Cheese Ravioli	Lean Cuisine	250
Pasta	Vermont Cheddar Mac & Cheese	Lean Cuisine	250
Pasta	Fettuccini Alfredo	Smart Ones	250
Poultry	Oriental Chicken	Smart Ones	250
Poultry	Fiesta Grilled Chicken	Lean Cuisine	250
Pasta	Chicken Linguini Red Pepper	Healthy Choice	250
Poultry	Golden Roasted Turkey Breast	Healthy Choice	250
Poultry	Chicken Mesquite	Smart Ones	250
Poultry	Chicken Oriental	Smart Ones	250
Poultry	Orange Sesame Chicken	Smart Ones	250
Poultry	Baked Chicken	Lean Cuisine	~~250~~ 260
Poultry	Teriyaki Chicken & Vegetables	Smart Ones	~~250~~ 260
Seafood	Tuna Noodle Casserole	Smart Ones	~~250~~ 270
Pasta	Spaghetti with Meatballs	Lean Cuisine	260
Poultry	Creamy Chicken & Noodles	Healthy Choice	260
Meat	Barbecue Steak with Red Potatoes	Healthy Choice	260

Pasta	Tortellini Primavera Parmesan	Healthy Choice	260
Pasta	Sesame Noodles with Vegetables	Smart Ones	260 280
Pasta	Creamy Rigatoni with Chicken	Smart Ones	260
Pasta	Macaroni & Cheese	Smart Ones	260
Pasta	Butternut Squash Ravioli	Lean Cuisine	260
Other	Santa Fe Rice & Beans	Smart Ones	260
Other	Coconut Chickpea Curry	Lean Cuisine	260
Poultry	Glazed Turkey Tenderloins	Lean Cuisine	270
Poultry	Kung Pao Chicken	Healthy Choice	270
Poultry	Chicken Margherita with Balsamic	Healthy Choice	270
Poultry	Chicken Strips & Sweet Potatoes	Smart Ones	270
Pasta	Spaghetti with Meat Sauce	Smart Ones	270 280
Meat	Salisbury Steak with Mac & Cheese	Lean Cuisine	270 290
Pasta	Penne Rosa	Lean Cuisine	270
Poultry	Turkey Breast & Stuffing	Smart Ones	270 280
Pasta	Classic Macaroni & Beef	Lean Cuisine	270
Pasta	Mushroom Mezzaluna Ravioli	Lean Cuisine	270
Pasta	Pasta with Swedish Meatballs	Smart Ones	280 290
Other	Asian Pot Stickers	Lean Cuisine	280
Poultry	Sesame Stir Fry with Chicken	Lean Cuisine	280
Poultry	Roasted Turkey Breast	Lean Cuisine	280 290
Poultry	Apple Cranberry Chicken	Lean Cuisine	280
Poultry	Chicken Fettuccini Alfredo	Healthy Choice	280
Poultry	Grilled Chicken Marinara	Healthy Choice	280
Poultry	Sweet & Spicy Orange Chicken	Healthy Choice	280
Poultry	Chicken Parmesan	Smart Ones	280
Poultry	Turkey Breast with Stuffing	Smart Ones	280
Meat	Beef & Broccoli	Healthy Choice	280
Meat	Meatball Marinara	Healthy Choice	280
Meat	Beef Teriyaki	Healthy Choice	280
Pasta	Spinach Artichoke Ravioli	Lean Cuisine	280

Entrée Type	Name	Brand	Calories
Pasta	Spinach Artichoke Ravioli	Lean Cuisine	280
Pasta	Linguini with Ricotta & Spinach	Lean Cuisine	280
Poultry	Chicken Fettuccini	Lean Cuisine	~~290~~ 280
Pasta	Spaghetti & Meatballs	Healthy Choice	280
Pasta	Spaghetti with Meat Sauce	Smart Ones	280
Other	Vegetable Fried Rice	Smart Ones	280
Other	Asian Pot Stickers	Lean Cuisine	280
Poultry	Chicken with Almonds	Lean Cuisine	290
Poultry	Chicken with Peanut Sauce	Lean Cuisine	290
Seafood	Shrimp & Angel Hair Pasta	Lean Cuisine	~~280~~ 290
Poultry	Grilled Chicken Pesto w Veggies	Healthy Choice	290
Poultry	General Tso's Spicy Chicken	Healthy Choice	290
Poultry	Pineapple Chicken	Healthy Choice	290
Poultry	Chicken Enchiladas Suiza	Smart Ones	290
Meat	Swedish Meatballs	Lean Cuisine	290
Seafood	Lemon Pepper Fish	Healthy Choice	290
Pasta	Pasta with Swedish Meatballs	Smart Ones	290
Other	Santa Fe Rice & Beans	Smart Ones	290
Pizza	Thin Crust Cheese Pizza	Smart Ones	290
Seafood	Parmesan Crusted Fish	Lean Cuisine	~~290~~ 300
Pasta	Santa Fe-Style Rice & Beans	Lean Cuisine	~~280~~ 300
Poultry	Roasted Turkey & Vegetables	Lean Cuisine	~~290~~ 300
Poultry	Sweet & Sour Chicken	Lean Cuisine	300
Poultry	Crustless Chicken Pot Pie	Healthy Choice	300
Poultry	Sweet Sesame Chicken	Healthy Choice	300
Poultry	Chicken Fettuccini	Smart Ones	300
Poultry	General Tso's Chicken	Smart Ones	300
Meat	Classic Meat Loaf	Healthy Choice	300
Seafood	Tortilla Crusted Fish	Lean Cuisine	~~300~~ 310
Pasta	Tuscan-Style Vegetable Lasagna	Lean Cuisine	~~300~~ 310

Entrée Type	Name	Brand	Calories
Pasta	Broccoli Cheddar Rotini	Lean Cuisine	300
Pasta	Three Cheese Ziti Marinara	Smart Ones	300
Pasta	Lasagna Florentine	Smart Ones	310 300
Seafood	Tortilla Crusted Fish	Lean Cuisine	300 310
Pasta	Tuscan-Style Vegetable Lasagna	Lean Cuisine	300 310
Poultry	Chicken Fried Rice	Lean Cuisine	300 310
Poultry	Orange Chicken	Lean Cuisine	310
Poultry	Chicken Tikka Masala	Lean Cuisine	310
Poultry	Chicken Strips & Fries	Smart Ones	310
Poultry	Chicken Teriyaki	Lean Cuisine	310
Pizza	Thin Crust Pepperoni Pizza	Smart Ones	310
Pasta	Three Cheese Macaroni	Smart Ones	310
Pizza	French Bread Pepperoni Pizza	Lean Cuisine	310
Poultry	Chicken Spinach Mushroom Panini	Lean Cuisine	350 310
Other	Spicy Beef & Bean Enchilada	Lean Cuisine	310
Poultry	Chicken Fried Rice	Healthy Choice	320
Meat	Sweet & Spicy Korean Beef	Lean Cuisine	320
Pizza	Farmers Market Pizza	Lean Cuisine	320
Pizza	Margherita Pizza	Lean Cuisine	320
Poultry	Chicken Carbonara	Lean Cuisine	330
Poultry	Mango Chicken w Coconut Rice	Lean Cuisine	330
Poultry	Country Fried Chicken	Healthy Choice	330
Other	Cheese & Fire-Roasted Tamale	Lean Cuisine	330
Poultry	Chicken Club Panini	Lean Cuisine	350 340
Meat	Philly Style Steak & Cheese Panini	Lean Cuisine	330 350
Poultry	Chicken Parmigiana	Healthy Choice	360
Poultry	Chicken Pecan	Lean Cuisine	320 370
Poultry	Sweet & Sour Chicken	Healthy Choice	390
Pizza	Supreme Pizza	Lean Cuisine	330 390

NoPaperPress eBooks and Paperbacks

100-Day Super Diet-1200 Cal*
100-Day Super Diet-1500 Cal*
100-Day No-Cooking Diet-1200 Cal*
100-Day No-Cooking Diet-1500 Cal*
90-Day Smart Diet-1200 Cal*
90-Day Smart Diet-1500 Cal*
90-Day No-Cooking Diet - 1200 Cal*
90-Day No-Cooking Diet - 1500 Cal*
90-Day Perfect Diet - 1200 Cal*
90-Day Perfect Diet - 1500 Cal*
60-Day Perfect Diet-1200 Cal*
60-Day Perfect Diet-1500 Cal*
50-Day Flex Diet-1200 Cal*
50-Day Flex Diet-1500 Cal*
30-Day Quick Diet - Women*
30-Day Quick Diet for Men*
30-Day No-Cooking Diet*
30-Day Diet for Women - Metric*
30-Day Diet for Men - Metric*
25 Day Easy Diet-1200 Cal*
25 Day Easy Diet-1500 Cal*
25-Day No-Cooking Diet
10-Day Express Diet
10-Day No-Cooking Diet*
7-Day Diet for Women*
7-Day Diet for Men*
7-Day No-Cooking Diets*
90-Day Gluten-Free Diet-1200 Cal*
90-Day Gluten-Free Diet-1500 Cal*
30-Day Gluten-Free Quick Diet*
30-Day Gluten-Free No-Cooking Diet*
7-Day Diet for Women - Metric*
7-Day Diet for Men - Metric
7-Day Gluten-Free Express Diet*
7-Day Gluten-Free No-Cooking Diet*
90-Day Vegetarian Diet-1200 Cal*
90-Day Vegetarian Diet-1500 Cal*
30-Day Vegetarian Diet*
7-Day Vegetarian Diet*
Weight Loss for Women*
Weight Loss for Women - Metric
Weight Loss for Women - UK
Weight Loss for Men*
Maximum Weight Loss - 1200 Cal*
Maximum Weight Loss - 1500 Cal*

Weight Loss for Men - Metric*
Maximum Weight Loss- 1200 Cal*
Maximum Weight Loss- 1500 Cal*
Weight Control - U.S. Edition*
Weight Control - Metric. Edition
Professional Weight Control Women - U.S.
Professional Weight Control Women - Metric
Professional Weight Control Men - U.S.
Professional Weight Control Men - Metric
Weight Maintenance - U.S. Ed*
Weight Maintenance - Metric. Ed*
Weight Maintenance - UK Ed
Weight Loss for Senior Men*
Weight Loss for Senior Women*
Eat Smart - U.S. Edition*
Eat Smart - Metric Edition
30-Day Mediterranean Diet
Exercise Smart - U.S. Edition*
Exercise Smart - Metric Edition
Exercise Smart - UK Edition*
Total Fitness - U.S. Edition
Total Fitness - Metric Edition
Total Fitness - UK Edition
Total Fitness for Women-U.S. Ed*
Total Fitness for Women - Metric
Total Fitness for Women - UK Ed
Total Fitness for Men - U.S. Ed*
Total Fitness for Men- Metric Ed*
Total Fitness for Men - UK Ed
Senior Fitness - U.S. Edition*
Senior Fitness - Metric Edition*
Senior Fitness - UK Edition*
Computer Diet - U.S. Edition*
Computer Diet - Metric Ed*
Reliable Weight Loss - U.S. Ed
101 Weight Loss Tips*
101 Healthy Eating Tips*
101 Lifelong Fitness Tips*
101 Weight Maintenance Tips
101 Weight Loss Recipes
101 GF Weight Loss Recipes
101 Veg Weight Loss Recipes*
30-Day Mediterranean Diet*
90-Day Med Diet - 1200 Cal*
90-Day Med Diet - 1500 Cal*

* These titles are available as both ebooks and paperbacks. Our ebooks are sold by Amazon, Apple, Google, Barnes & Noble and Kobo, but our paperbacks are only sold by Amazon.